S0-CDW-940

Fine Needle Aspiration of Subcutaneous Organs and Masses

Fine Needle Aspiration of Subcutaneous Organs and Masses

Editors

YENER S. EROZAN, M.D.
Professor, Department of Pathology
Division of Cytopathology
The Johns Hopkins University
Baltimore, Maryland

THOMAS A. BONFIGLIO, M.D.
Professor and Chair
Pathologist-in-Chief
Department of Pathology and Laboratory Medicine
University of Rochester
Rochester, New York

RC 270.3
N44
F56
1996

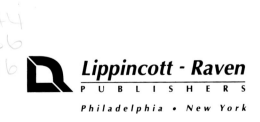

Lippincott - Raven
PUBLISHERS
Philadelphia • New York

Acquisitions Editor: Vickie E. Thaw
Senior Developmental Editor: Judith E. Hummel
Project Editor: Carolyn A. Kuehn
Production Manager: Caren Erlichman
Production Coordinator: David Yurkovich
Design Coordinator: Doug Smock
Indexer: Holly C. Lukens
Compositor: Tapsco, Inc.
Printer: Mandarin Offset

Printed in Hong Kong

Copyright © 1996 by Lippincott–Raven Publishers.

All rights reserved. This book is protected by copyright. No part of it may be
reproduced, stored in a retrieval system, or transmitted, in any form or by any
means—electronic, mechanical, photocopy, recording, or otherwise—without the
prior written permission of the publisher, except for brief quotations embodied in
critical articles and reviews. For information write Lippincott–Raven Publishers,
227 East Washington Square, Philadelphia, PA 19106.

Materials appearing in this book prepared by individuals as part of their official
duties as U.S. Government employees are not covered by the above-mentioned
copyright.

Library of Congress Cataloging-in-Publication Data

Fine needle aspiration of subcutaneous organs and masses/editors,
    Yener S. Erozan, Thomas A. Bonfiglio.—1st ed.
        p. cm.
    Includes bibliographical references and index.
    ISBN 0-397-51502-2 (alk. paper)
    1. Tumors—Needle biopsy. 2. Breast—Needle biopsy. 3. Salivary
glands—Needle Biopsy. 4. Lymph nodes—Needle biopsy. 5. Thyroid
gland—Needle Biopsy. I. Erozan, Yener S. II. Bonfiglio, Thomas A.
    [DNLM: 1. Biospy, Needle. WB 379 F4953 1996]
RC270.3.N44F56   1996
616.07′582—dc20
DNLM/DLC
for Library of Congress   96-6217
                                                                  CIP

Care has been taken to confirm the accuracy of the information presented and to
describe generally accepted practices. However, the authors, editors, and publisher
are not responsible for errors or omissions or for any consequences from application
of the information in this book and make no warranty, express or implied, with
respect to the contents of the publication.
    The authors, editors, and publisher have exerted every effort to ensure that drug
selection and dosage set forth in this text are in accordance with current
recommendations and practice at the time of publication. However, in view of
ongoing research, changes in government regulations, and the constant flow of
information relating to drug therapy and drug reactions, the reader is urged to check
the package insert for each drug for any change in indications and dosage and for
added warnings and precautions. This is particularly important when the
recommended agent is a new or infrequently employed drug.
    Some drugs and medical devices presented in this publication have Food and
Drug Administration (FDA) clearance for limited use in restricted research settings.
It is the responsibility of the health care provider to ascertain the FDA status of each
drug or device planned for use in their clinical practice.

9 8 7 6 5 4 3 2 1

To our wives, Brenda and Mary

Contributor List

Wendie A. Berg, M.D., Ph.D., *Assistant Professor, Chief of Breast Imaging, Department of Diagnostic Radiology, University of Maryland Medical System, 22 South Greene Street, Baltimore, MD 21201*

Thomas A. Bonfiglio, M.D., *Professor and Chair, Pathologist-in-Chief, Department of Pathology and Laboratory Medicine, University of Rochester, 601 Elmwood Avenue, Box 626, Rochester, NY 14642*

Anne E. Busseniers, M.D., *Medical Director, Metropolitan Aspiration Clinic, 1850 Town Center Parkway, Suite 407, Reston, VA 22090*

Nancy P. Caraway, M.D., *Assistant Professor, Department of Pathology, The University of Texas, M.D. Anderson Cancer Center, Section of Cytology, 1515 Holcombe Boulevard, Box 53, Houston, TX 77030*

Andrea E. Dawson, M.D., *Associate Professor, University of Rochester Medical Center, Department of Pathology and Laboratory Medicine, Surgical Pathology Unit, 601 Elmwood Avenue, Rochester, NY 14642*

Yener S. Erozan, M.D., *Professor of Pathology, Department of Pathology, Division of Cytopathology, The Johns Hopkins University, 600 North Wolfe Street, Baltimore, MD 21287-6940*

John R. Goellner, M.D., *Consultant, Division of Anatomic Pathology, Mayo Clinic and Mayo Foundation, Geraldine Colby Zeiler Professor of Cytopathology, Mayo Medical School, 200 First Street, SW, Rochester, MN 55905*

Ruth L. Katz, M.D., *Professor of Pathology, Co-Chief, Section of Cytology, Department of Pathology, The University of Texas, M.D. Anderson Cancer Center, 1515 Holcombe Boulevard, Box 53, Houston, TX 77030*

Dina R. Mody, M.D., *Associate Medical Director of Cytology, The Methodist Hospital, Associate Professor of Pathology, Department of Pathology, Baylor College of Medicine, One Baylor Plaza, Houston, TX 77030*

Ibrahim Ramzy, M.D., *Chief, Anatomic Pathology, The Methodist Hospital, Professor of Pathology and Obstetrics-Gynecology, Baylor College of Medicine, One Baylor Plaza, Houston, TX 77030*

H. Rosy Singh, M.D., *Assistant Professor, Department of Radiology, Johns Hopkins Outpatient Center, Breast Imaging Center, 601 North Caroline Street, Baltimore, MD 21287*

Introduction

There are many monographs, specialized books, and texts currently available in the field of diagnostic cytopathology. Even so, we feel there is a need and a place for a new set of publications in the field. Using the traditional cytologic approaches of The University of Rochester and The Johns Hopkins Laboratories, our vision is to publish a series of text-atlases that emphasizes current diagnostic criteria, uses modern terminology, and looks to the future of this rapidly evolving subspecialty of pathology.

Because the emphasis is on useful and practical diagnostic criteria, we devised a format that uses many more illustrations than most standard texts. Although descriptive text is essential, the available vocabulary is limited; more figures are necessary to adequately detail the many possible and variable nuances of cytologic features that are often seen within a single diagnostic category. This design will, we hope, provide the reader with both a better appreciation of the morphologic features that the authors discuss and a useful reference to help solve routine differential diagnostic problems encountered in the typical cytopathology practice.

Yener S. Erozan, M.D.
Thomas A. Bonfiglio, M.D.

Preface

The use of fine needle aspiration (FNA) for cytopathologic diagnosis of neoplasms and nonneoplastic diseases of subcutaneous organs and tissues has recently increased in popularity in the United States. It is a challenging area for pathologists, not only because of the microscopic interpretation but also because of the performance of the procedure.

The optimal cytopathologic diagnosis depends on proper specimen collection and preparation; without these, microscopic interpretation becomes a futile effort. Chapter 1 of *Fine Needle Aspiration of Subcutaneous Organs and Masses* is devoted to FNA technique and preparation of the aspirates. Another role of the pathologist is to assist the radiologist in obtaining optimal specimens during radiologically guided FNAs. Although radiologic guidance is of limited use in subcutaneous FNAs, it is important in the diagnosis of nonpalpable breast lesions and certain thyroid lesions. The effectiveness of this technique and its applications are briefly presented in Chapter 2.

The aim of this book is to give readers well-illustrated presentations of cytopathologic findings in fine needle aspirates of subcutaneous lesions and to offer guidance for approaching diagnostic problems and avoiding mistakes. The use of ancillary techniques (eg, immunochemistry and flow cytometry) is also discussed in appropriate areas.

In books by multiple authors, some overlap of subjects and some differences of opinion are unavoidable. These, however, probably help to achieve the purpose of this book.

Yener S. Erozan, M.D.
Thomas A. Bonfiglio, M.D.

Contents

Fine Needle Aspiration
of Subcutaneous
Organs and Masses

● ●

Fine Needle Aspiration of Subcutaneous Organs and Masses,
edited by Yener S. Erozan and Thomas A. Bonfiglio.
Lippincott–Raven Publishers, Philadelphia, © 1996.

CHAPTER 1

Superficial Fine Needle Aspiration

Introduction and Technique

Anne E. Busseniers

Striving for containment of medical costs has resulted in the development and application of cost-effective and less invasive yet accurate diagnostic procedures. Fine needle aspiration (FNA) of superficial and deep-seated lesions has emerged as one such tool.[1-6] Continual refinement of cytologic criteria as well as availability and application of ancillary studies on smaller tissue samples have improved the sensitivity and specificity of the technique for most body sites.

A successful approach to FNA is one that combines the following factors:

1. The procedure is performed by an experienced physician skilled in palpation, who has mastered the technique and is convinced of its usefulness and performs an adequate number of aspirations to keep up his or her skill.
2. The sample is adequate, representative, and microscopically interpretable.
3. The patient is comfortable at all times.
4. An accurate diagnosis is available in a timely fashion.

5. The material is interpreted by a pathologist with special interest and training in cytopathology.

This chapter describes the basic collection technique of FNA of superficial, palpable masses, used at The Johns Hopkins Hospital. In many ways, it is similar to the one previously described by Oertel.[7]

WHO SHOULD PERFORM THE ASPIRATION?

This issue remains controversial. In our experience, the best results are obtained when FNA is performed by a trained cytopathologist as an outpatient procedure in a specially prepared room, preferably within the cytopathology laboratory. The advantages of this system are multiple:

1. A limited number of individuals consistently gain experience instead of diffusing the expertise among physicians of various specialties.
2. Physicians from any specialty interested in learning the procedure can be trained under the supervision of the cytopathologist. This guarantees uniformity in technique and smear preparation.

A. E. Busseniers: Medical Director, Metropolitan Aspiration Clinic, Reston, VA 22090.

3. Optimal smear preparation is enhanced by the assistance of an experienced technologist.

4. Immediate evaluation of the material provides for increased sample adequacy, because the procedure can be repeated while the patient is still in the office, and provides for increased accuracy by allowing allocation of material for ancillary studies. Finally, the preliminary results, which are often the final interpretation, are available to clinicians in a timely fashion and permit early patient counseling and initiation of therapy.

5. Results of a targeted clinical history, physical examination, and radiologic studies, as well as the gross appearance of the aspirated material are readily available; all aid in arriving at the correct diagnosis.

ANCILLARY PERSONNEL

An FNA coordinator is recommended to schedule patients and to obtain the necessary information for billing. At our institution, this is a technologist who has the first contact with the patient over the telephone and at the time of FNA. The coordinator fills out the necessary paperwork, is trained to give a brief explanation of the procedure, and assists the pathologist with the FNA.

A technologist who is familiar with the equipment, the procedure, various smearing techniques, and staining and who has experience in patient contact is best able to achieve optimal results.

SPACE AND EQUIPMENT

The aspiration room should be equipped with the following: adequate lighting; a comfortable examination table; a curtain for privacy when the patient undresses; and adequate counter space with a sink and storage area for stains, equipment, and supplies. It also should include a desk with a microscope located separately from the patient area, where the cytopathologist reviews slides for specimen adequacy and may, in privacy, obtain additional clinical information from the referring physicians.

The equipment is simple and includes, among other things, a syringe holder: we prefer the 10-mL syringe holder over the 20-mL syringe holder because it is less bulky and limits the distance between the target and the aspirator's hand, allowing for more stability. We use disposable 10-mL syringes with Luer-Lok tip. Also needed are needles with clear hub. We routinely use the following sizes: 22 gauge 1 inch long, 22 gauge 1 1/2 inch long, 23 gauge 1 inch long, and 25 gauge. The size of the lesion to be sampled and its estimated depth dictate the size and length of the needle. Other items include alcohol-soaked swabs and gauze pads, plastic slide holders to align the glass slides, glass slides with one frosted end used for labeling, a hemocytometer cover glass used to smear the material, 95% alcohol for wet-fixed smears, a balanced solution for cell-block preparation from needle rinses, and gloves, ammonia, and an ice pack.

THE PATIENT

The patient is greeted and the members of the aspiration team are introduced. It takes time to prepare a patient mentally for the procedure. Spending a few minutes discussing issues not related to the procedure helps relax the patient as long as the team is sincere and genuinely caring.

A targeted clinical history and physical examination is obtained. Radiographs or results from related radiologic studies, if available, should be reviewed to confirm the clinical impression and the location of the mass.

The procedure is explained in basic terms with emphasis on its simplicity and safety. We routinely compare the FNA procedure with a venipuncture and stress that the needles used for FNA are smaller than the ones used for drawing blood. We explain that an average of three passes are performed to obtain a representative sample of the lesion. The patient is given ample opportunity to ask questions, and informed consent is obtained.

Palpation of the mass to evaluate its size and depth and proper positioning of the patient are essential. Finding a position that is comfortable for the patient, usually supine or slightly upright, and optimal for the aspirator is the first crucial step toward sampling the correct area. With a small lesion, these steps usually take more time than the FNA itself.

TECHNIQUE

The lesion is immobilized between the second and third fingers of the left hand (for a right-handed aspirator), leaving the thumb free to guide or support the aspiration device (Figs. 1-1 and 1-2).

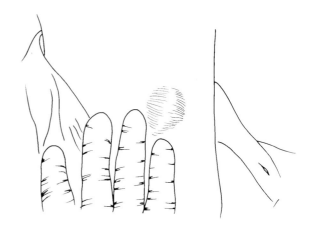

FIG. 1-1. The mass is immobilized between the second and third fingers.

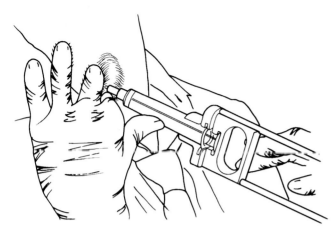

FIG. 1-2. The thumb of the hand used to immobilize the lesion supports and guides the aspiration device.

The skin is cleaned with an alcohol-soaked swab and dried with gauze, or the alcohol is allowed to evaporate. Any alcohol left on the skin will produce unnecessary pain when the needle is inserted.

The assistant prepares and hands the equipment to the cytopathologist step by step. We have found it very useful to have the assistant hold the patient's hand while the procedure is being done. Hand-holding is our substitute for an anesthetic. Discomfort experienced by patients with a low tolerance for pain can be diminished by applying a small ice pack on the puncture site after the first pass. This numbs the skin and facilitates additional passes.

Aspiration Technique Using the Syringe Holder

A small amount of air is aspirated into the syringe, and the needle is subsequently guided into the lesion, usually perpendicular to the skin surface. A variable amount of suction is applied by pulling the plunger back, while a

vigorous vertical and slightly circular movement is made to "dislodge" the cells and tissue fragments (Fig. 1-3). This vigorous to-and-fro motion is done in the same plane, not in a fanlike fashion. Close attention is paid to the nature and amount of the material appearing in the needle hub. The material should remain within the hub, and when it becomes bloody, the procedure should be interrupted.

The suction is released before withdrawing the needle. If this step is omitted, the material will invariably be aspirated into the barrel of the syringe. It may then be retrieved by rinsing in a balanced salt solution for subsequent cell-block preparation.

Nonaspiration Technique

The needle is attached to the syringe and the plunger removed. Cleaning of the skin is done as described earlier. The aspiration device is held as one would hold a pencil, the needle is inserted into the lesion, and the material is dislodged from the mass through rapid, vigorous, back-and-forth movements (Fig. 1-4). This technique allows the proximal part of the aspirator's hand to rest on the patient's body, which improves stability. The technique also enhances difference in texture, allowing more accurate placement of the needle, particularly in small lesions. To prepare the smears, the plunger is once again inserted into the barrel.

Three passes are routinely performed to sample a mass of average size. For each pass, the needle is inserted into a different area of the lesion, usually the upper, middle, and lower regions.

Pressure is applied with a clean gauze pad at the needle site after each pass to prevent the development of a local hematoma. If a hematoma develops, additional passes are nearly impossible to perform. The hematoma may become quite substantial, which usually is the result of

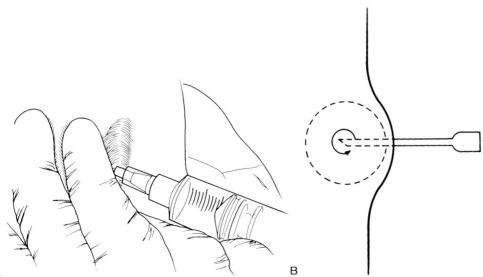

A   B

FIG. 1-3. (A) As soon as the needle is inserted into the lesion, the plunger is pulled back to allow for a small amount of suction, usually around 2 to 3 mL. **(B)** The needle is moved back and forth vigorously while small circular movements are made in the same plane.

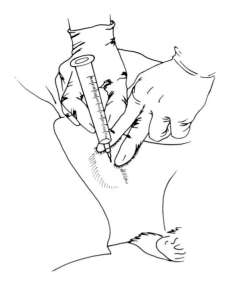

FIG. 1-4. For the nonaspiration technique, the position of the fingers used to immobilize the mass is similar to that in the aspiration technique. The syringe with attached needle is held as one would hold a pencil, while the proximal part of the hand rests on the patient.

inadequate supervision. The patient should be instructed to push on the puncture site, and the physician should check the area as soon as the smears are made.

Some patients or an accompanying family member may become light-headed and faint. It is best to perform the first pass with the patient in the supine position and have a small vial of ammonia at hand.

The smears are made as soon as possible to avoid clotting of the material. The procedure can be repeated as many times as is dictated by the immediate evaluation.

PREPARATION OF THE SMEARS

The slides and hemocytometer cover glass should be prepared in advance to avoid delay in smearing. A small amount of material is dropped close to the frosted edge of several slides (Fig. 1-5).

Solid masses usually yield enough material to prepare two to six smears. In case of cystic or bloody fluid, we routinely prepare four direct smears and submit the rest for cytospin (cyst fluid) or cell-block preparation (bloody material).

Care should be taken to turn the bevel of the needle toward the slide. This avoids the splashing of material if a little resistance is encountered when expelling the material.

The smears are prepared as a peripheral blood smear using the hemocytometer cover glass (Fig. 1-6). This technique minimizes crushing artifact and concentrates the cells and tissue fragments on the interpretable portions of the glass slide.

Visible tissue fragments can be gently crushed to produce a monolayer, or they may be removed and included with the needle rinses to be processed as a small biopsy.

If the material is semisolid (eg, abundant colloid, mucin), it is best smeared by holding the hemocytometer cover glass parallel to the glass slide and smearing the material in a fanlike fashion (Fig. 1-7). We use a combination of air-dried, Diff-Quik–stained and alcohol-fixed, Papanicolaou-stained, or hematoxylin–eosin-stained material.

Our needle rinses are not routinely processed. The rinses will not yield much additional information when the smears are paucicellular. If the preliminary evaluation reveals that the diagnosis will be more accurately made by histologic evaluation, we routinely perform additional passes from which the entire material is submitted for cell-block preparation.

COMMONLY ASKED QUESTIONS

Is It Necessary to Use an Anesthetic?

We perform FNA without local anesthesia. Injecting the anesthetic under the skin is painful for the patient and may require more than one needle stick. Although the anesthetic numbs the skin, a considerable amount of pain may still be felt by the patient during the procedure. More importantly, the anesthetic may render small nodules, such as lymph nodes, difficult to palpate by creating an artificial superimposed mass. Furthermore, a specimen diluted by the anesthetic solution may destroy the cells and render the sample uninterpretable. A patient who has been mentally prepared by good communication and verbal comforting and who is adequately guided through the procedure does not require an anesthetic. As an alternative, one can use a small ice pack that the patient is instructed to hold over the mass for a few minutes.

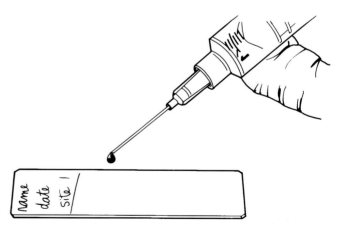

FIG. 1-5. A small amount of aspirated material is dropped on the glass slide close to the frosted end.

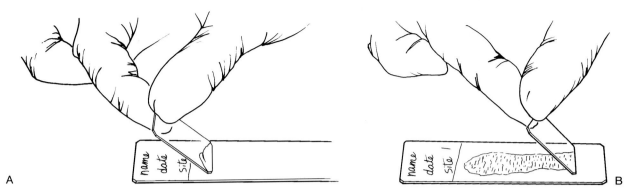

FIG. 1-6. The aspirated material is spread on the glass slide using a hemocytometer cover glass, as is done in the preparation of a peripheral blood smear.

How Much Suction?

The appropriate amount of suction depends on the mass to be sampled. Thyroid lesions generally require no more than 3 to 4 mL of suction if the aspiration method is used. Additional suction may be required if the lesion is fibrotic, as in long-standing chronic lymphocytic thyroiditis or papillary carcinoma. Benign breast lesions often require full 10-mL suction as well as more prolonged and vigorous vertical movements before material appears in the needle hub. Applying gradual suction and observing the needle hub for the appearance of material determines the amount of suction needed.

Why Vertical and Slightly Circular Movements?

Vertical movement during a pass produces trauma to the tissue in only one direction. If the aspiration is performed using a fanlike movement, increased tearing of the tissue produces more hemorrhage, damages adjacent tissue, and limits the yield of additional passes. Small cir-

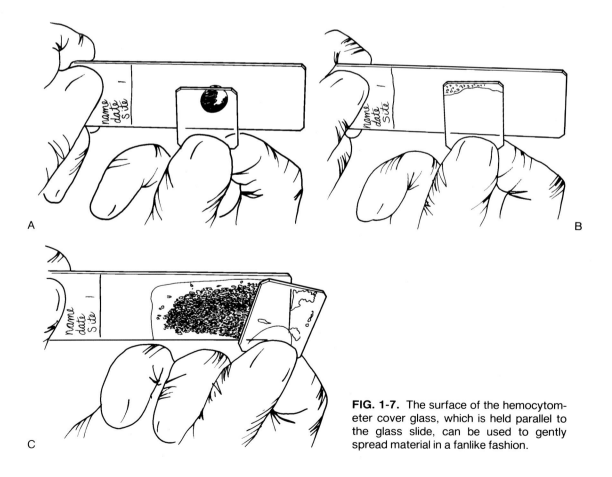

FIG. 1-7. The surface of the hemocytometer cover glass, which is held parallel to the glass slide, can be used to gently spread material in a fanlike fashion.

cular movements help to dislodge material and are best thought of as scraping the inside of the lesion with the bevel of the needle.

Aspiration or Nonaspiration Technique?

The aspiration device provides stability and allows one free hand to immobilize the mass, factors particularly important for relatively small masses (ie, those less than 2 cm). By preventing the mass from moving during the aspiration, one increases the accuracy of placement of the needle. Immobilization also permits better control of the amount of suction needed and generally yields larger tissue fragments. We use the nonaspiration technique for superficial and very small lesions (less than 1 cm).

Can Fine Needle Aspiration Be Performed When the Patient Is on Anticoagulation Therapy?

The size of the needles used for superficial FNA is sufficiently small that extraordinary bleeding is not usually experienced.

Is There a Risk of Infection?

Although we include the risk of infection as a possible side effect of FNA in our informed consent form, we have not observed this occurrence in any of our patients.

COMMON MISTAKES

Common mistakes include not spending enough time to prepare the patient mentally, not spending enough time to find the optimal position for palpation and immobilization of the lesion, and not drying the skin before inserting the needle. Technical mistakes include pulling the plunger to the full 10 mL mark, pumping the plunger instead of moving the needle, not using vigorous back-and-forth motion to dislodge the material, forgetting to release suction before withdrawing the needle from the lesion, not applying pressure at the puncture site with resulting hematoma, and allowing material to clot before making the smears.

REFERENCES

1. Brown LA, Coghill SB. Cost effectiveness of a fine needle aspiration clinic. Cytopathology 1992;3:278.
2. Kaminsky DB. Aspiration biopsy in the context of the new medicare fiscal policy. Acta Cytol 1984;28:333.
3. Layfield LJ, Chrischilles EA, Cohen MB, et al. The palpable breast nodule: a cost-effectiveness analysis of alternate diagnostic approaches. Cancer 1993;72:1642.
4. Oertel YC, Zorsky PE. Fine needle aspiration as a means to cost-effective health care. South Med J 1993;86:282.
5. Paotella LP, Cronan JJ, Dorfman GS, et al. Dollars and sense of percutaneous biopsy. Rhode Island Med J 1987;70:127.
6. Smith TJ, Sofaii H, Foster EA, et al. Accuracy and cost-effectiveness of fine needle aspiration biopsy. Am J Surg 1985;149:540.
7. Oertel YC. Fine needle aspiration: a personal view. Lab Med 1982;13:343.

Fine Needle Aspiration of Subcutaneous Organs and Masses,
edited by Yener S. Erozan and Thomas A. Bonfiglio.
Lippincott–Raven Publishers, Philadelphia, © 1996.

CHAPTER 2

Imaging-Guided Fine Needle Aspiration of Breast, Thyroid, and Subcutaneous Masses

Wendie A. Berg and H. Rosy Singh

FINE NEEDLE ASPIRATION OF BREAST LESIONS

Screening mammography has considerably improved detection of breast cancer, but it has also led to the excision of many benign lesions. Because only 15% to 30% of mammographically suspicious abnormalities prove to be malignant,[1–3] increasing attention is being given to nonsurgical biopsy methods. These methods include fine needle aspiration (FNA), typically performed with a 22- to 25-gauge needle, and large core needle biopsy, using a 14-gauge needle, under ultrasound or stereotactic mammographic guidance. Using such methods, the number of open surgical biopsies for benign disease can be substantially reduced,[4–7] and patients with a malignant needle biopsy can undergo a single therapeutic surgical procedure. Similarly, a definitively benign needle biopsy reduces the need for short-term mammographic follow-up and alleviates patient anxiety.

Breast lesions usually become apparent through screening mammography or the discovery of a palpable mass. In either case, it is imperative to thoroughly evaluate a bilateral mammogram, because breast cancer is multicentric in 30% to 45% of cases of invasive breast cancer at presentation[8] and bilateral in 3% to 5% of cases.

Conversely, an unremarkable mammogram should not preclude biopsy of a clinically suspicious mass; Edeiken[9] found that of 499 patients with palpable carcinomas, 108 (22%) had falsely normal mammograms. Overall, mammography misses about 9% of breast cancers.[1]

Ultrasound is used to characterize mammographically well-defined or clinically palpable masses. The most common breast mass is the simple cyst. Cysts are particularly common in premenopausal women and those on hormone replacement therapy, usually resolve spontaneously,[10] and generally do not require aspiration. Using ultrasound criteria, a simple cyst is an anechoic mass that has a well-defined back wall and enhanced through transmission (Fig. 2-1).

If internal echoes exist or if a mural nodule is detected on ultrasound, aspiration and pneumocystography are appropriate. Fortunately, fewer than 1% of breast cancers occur as intracystic masses (Fig. 2-2). Pneumocystography, which involves the injection of a small amount of air into the cyst followed by repeat mammography, is also advocated in the evaluation of recurrent breast cysts[11,12] because small mural nodules may become evident. As a side benefit, injection of a small amount of air into a simple cyst has been reported to decrease the incidence of recurrence.[13] If a cyst becomes very large or painful, aspiration may be considered on clinical grounds.

An aspirate of clear or cloudy tan to bluish-green fluid from a cyst can safely be dismissed as benign and does not merit cytologic analysis. In a study of 6782 consecutive breast fluids, Ciatto and colleagues[14] found that 2%

  W. A. Berg: Department of Diagnostic Radiology, University of Maryland Medical System, Baltimore, MD 21201.
  H. R. Singh: Department of Radiology, Johns Hopkins Outpatient Center, Baltimore, MD 21287.

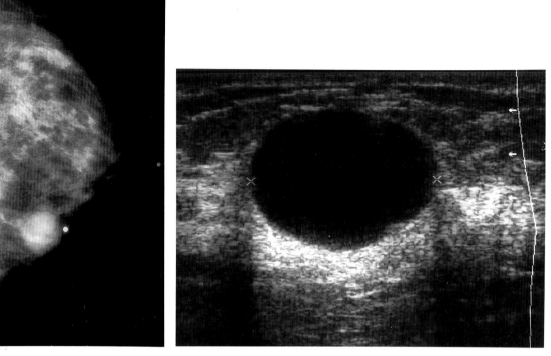

FIG. 2-1. Mammogram and ultrasound of a simple cyst. This 53-year-old woman presented with a palpable mass in the right breast. **(A)** Craniocaudal mammogram shows a B-B on the circumscribed mass (*white dot*) in the inner right breast equal in density to the surrounding parenchyma. **(B)** Ultrasound shows the mass to be anechoic with enhanced through transmission and a well-defined back wall compatible with a simple cyst. No further intervention is needed.

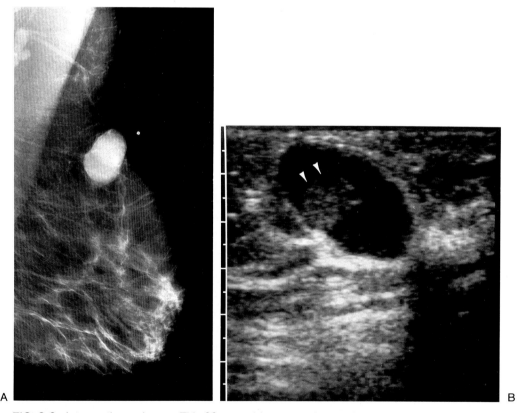

FIG. 2-2. Intracystic carcinoma. This 66-year-old woman observed a palpable mass in the right breast. **(A)** Mediolateral oblique mammogram shows a B-B on the dense circumscribed mass (*white dot*) in the upper right breast. **(B)** Ultrasound demonstrated a hypoechoic mural mass (*arrows*) in this case of intracystic papillary carcinoma. A 6-mm infiltrating ductal carcinoma was also found immediately adjacent to the intracystic carcinoma.

of aspirates were bloody: all 5 cases of intracystic papilloma and 1 case of lobular carcinoma in situ had bloody fluid and showed intracystic masses at pneumocystography. Even in these cases, cytology of the bloody fluid was unreliable; such cases merit close follow-up.

Aspiration is the most appropriate next step in the evaluation of the sonographically indeterminate mass, that is, a mass that is hypoechoic on ultrasound with enhanced through transmission (Fig. 2-3) or one which is anechoic with no enhanced through transmission. These lesions frequently prove to be hemorrhagic cysts. A needle with a larger bore, such as an 18-gauge needle, is sometimes needed with such lesions to aspirate fluid that may be unusually viscous. Cysts that are 5 mm or smaller can lack definitive sonographic criteria for a simple cyst; management in these cases should be predicated on the mammographic appearance.

If a mass is solid, the alternatives are imaging follow-up (mammography or ultrasound) or biopsy. For masses with irregular or indistinct margins, needle biopsy or excisional biopsy should be performed. In the case of a circumscribed mass of any size, the risk of malignancy is sufficiently low (1.4%) that radiologic follow-up is usually considered appropriate.[15,16] However, because the greatest treatment successes are in cancers that are smaller than 1 cm at diagnosis, and because nonsurgical biopsy and FNA are inexpensive, some advocate FNA as an alternative to short-term follow-up of probably benign lesions.[17,18]

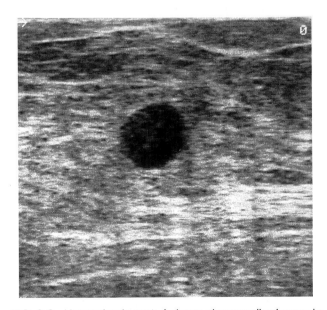

FIG. 2-3. Hemorrhagic cyst. A dense circumscribed mass in the upper outer left breast was detected on a screening mammogram of this 70-year-old woman. Ultrasound revealed a well-defined mass with internal echoes. Aspiration yielded bloody fluid that was sent for cytopathologic analysis, and the result was benign, compatible with a hemorrhagic cyst.

Methods

Obtaining an adequate sample with FNA is of primary importance, with insufficient sample rates ranging from 0.1% to 45%.[19] A strict definition of an adequate sample is lacking, but most cytopathologists require four to six clusters of at least six ductal epithelial cells on two or more smears. Several factors affect specimen quality, including the experience of both the person performing the procedure and the cytopathologist interpreting the smears, the nature of the lesion, the accuracy of needle placement, the number of samples obtained, and the processing of the specimen. Representative material was more often obtained in several series when the pathologist performed the procedure[19,20] or was at least present, permitting on-site evaluation with additional passes directed to areas of interest. A review of 13,066 cases of FNA performed across multiple institutions revealed a mean frequency of unsatisfactory aspirates of 18% when performed by nonpathologists, compared with 7.2% when performed by pathologists.[21] Appropriate placement of the needle must be confirmed. For nonpalpable lesions, FNA can be performed with the guidance of a mammographic grid (as is used in needle localization for excisional biopsy), with stereotactic guidance, or with ultrasound guidance. Because the depth is not as precisely controlled in the case of the grid, results are less often diagnostic with this method.[22,23] With stereotactic guidance (Fig. 2-4), the lesion must have satisfactory conspicuity on two stereo images, taken at 30 degrees to each other, and must be accessible (ie, not too superficial or too close to the chest wall). The nature of the lesion and the density of the breast can affect the ability to obtain an adequate sample. A dense breast can adversely affect lesion conspicuity and alter the course of the needle. Similarly, a firm lesion, such as a fibroadenoma, within a fatty breast may be displaced by the needle.

Many investigators prefer ultrasound guidance for its relative ease of patient and lesion positioning and setup.[24,25] No radiation exposure is needed, and superficial lesions can be more easily targeted. Mammographic (stereotactic) guidance is still required for microcalcifications; overall, only about half of mammographically detected lesions are visible sonographically.[26]

A variety of methods for preparation of the smears and fixation techniques have been proposed. In the traditional method, a 10- or 20-mL syringe is connected directly or by tubing to a 22- or 23-gauge needle. After infiltration of the skin with 1% lidocaine, the needle is advanced, and needle position within the lesion is confirmed (Fig. 2-5; see Fig. 2-4). A syringe holder can be used to create a vacuum, and about 10 quick 1-cm excursion passes are made through the lesion (until material is observed in the hub of the needle). Suction is then released, the needle is removed, and smears are made as described later. If blood is obtained, aspiration should be

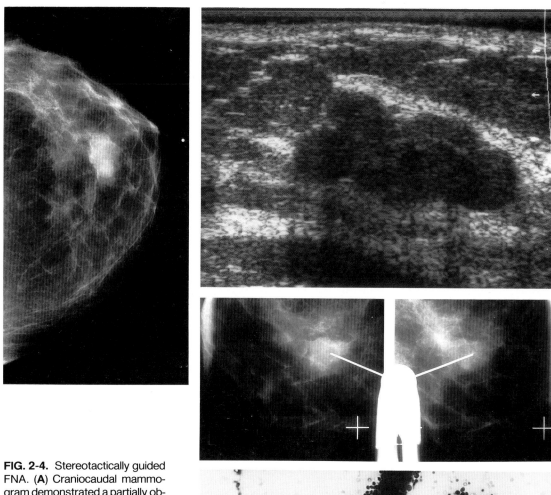

FIG. 2-4. Stereotactically guided FNA. **(A)** Craniocaudal mammogram demonstrated a partially obscured lobulated mass in the central portion of the right breast in this 38-year-old asymptomatic woman. **(B)** Ultrasound revealed a circumscribed hypoechoic lobulated mass. **(C)** Stereotactic images obtained immediately before FNA with the breast in compression (Fischer Mammotest Unit, Fischer Imaging Corporation, Denver, CO), each taken at 15 degrees off axis, demonstrate successful placement of the 22-gauge needle within the center of the mass. **(D)** Diff-Quik–stained cytology specimen shows the typical "antler horn" configuration of ductal-type epithelium with myoepithelial cells characteristic for a fibroadenoma. (×40)

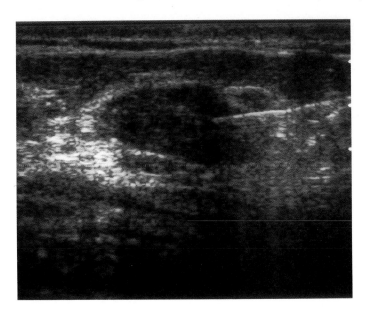

FIG. 2-5. Ultrasound-guided FNA. Under direct sonographic visualization, using a 7.5-MHz linear array transducer, FNA was performed on a hypoechoic, well-defined mass, which proved to be a fibroadenoma.

discontinued because it is detrimental to specimen quality.

The number of samples obtained can affect specimen adequacy. Diagnostic yield has been shown to improve when at least three aspirates are obtained from the lesion. In a study by Patel and associates,[27] the sensitivity for detection of malignancy was 64% for the first aspiration and 91% in patients who had three aspirates. Similar results were obtained by Pennes and coworkers,[28] who demonstrated incremental diagnostic yields for additional passes and extrapolated that 10 passes would be needed to achieve 100% sensitivity. The capillary technique, wherein no suction is applied, tends to yield superior quality material, with cellular yields comparable to[29] or slightly less than traditional FNA.[30]

A number of methods for slide preparation have been described. Many investigators place one drop of material on a slide, invert a second slide over the drop, and as the material spreads, pull the two slides apart horizontally. The *book-opening* or *vertical* technique[31] has been reported to yield superior material with less air drying and smear artifact[32] than the horizontal technique. In the former method, gentle pressure is applied to the upper slide, resulting in a 1- to 2-cm diameter specimen, and the slides are turned apart without pulling. One slide is then air dried and stained with modified Wright, Diff-Quik, or Romanovsky stain, and the second slide is immediately fixed in 95% ethanol for Papanicolaou staining. Three to five drops of material are anticipated per aspirate (yielding 6 to 10 slides). Paraffin-embedded cell blocks can also be prepared from washings of the needle in Hanks balanced salt solution or Cytolite. The latter technique is preferred for immunoperoxidase studies. Estrogen receptor and progesterone receptor content can be accurately quantified from such cytologic specimens.[33–35] Prognostic factors such as DNA ploidy[36] and nuclear grade[37] can also be determined on cytologic specimens.

Results

The most important goal in FNA is detection and exclusion of malignancy (Fig. 2-6). FNA is effective if physicians adhere to strict criteria of acceptable specimens and adequate sampling. Reported sensitivities range from 65% to 98%, and specificities range from 34% to 100%.[12,21,38,39] In determining sensitivity, many studies include cases deemed suspicious as positive results; across multiple series in which all patients had histologic correlation,[4,40–45] 92% of suspicious lesions proved to be malignant (Table 2-1).

The results of published series are difficult to compare for several reasons. Many studies have dismissed nondiagnostic and acellular aspirates as probably benign without excisional proof. Their exclusion from the data falsely improves the specificity, sensitivity, and accuracy of the procedure. Table 2-1 illustrates that in most series in which all patients underwent excision, cancers were missed in the nondiagnostic group. Overall in these studies, 38 of 409 insufficient samples (9.3%) proved to be malignant. Some studies include cysts among the benign lesions. As previously discussed, these could have been distinguished from solid lesions by aspiration alone, without the need for cytology.

In cases of mammographically or clinically suspicious lesions and a benign, atypical, or nondiagnostic cytopathologic result, repeat aspiration or excisional biopsy should be performed. Excisional biopsy of every *atypical* fine needle aspirate results in unnecessary biopsies; some advocate mammographic and clinical follow-up of the clinically or mammographically benign lesion with atypical cytology.[44] However, the rate of malignancy in specimens with atypia varies from 0% to 49% (see Table 2-1). In a review of 1181 consecutive abnormal cytopathology reports correlated with the mammographic and clinical impressions, Ciatto and colleagues[45] reported that the

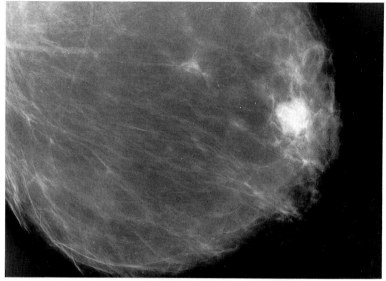

A

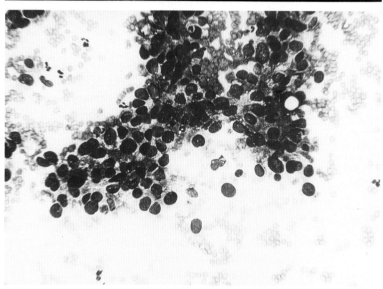

B

FIG. 2-6. Infiltrating ductal cancer. (A) Mammo-gram shows a partially indistinct lobulated mass in the retroareolar area of the right breast in this 51-year-old asymptomatic woman. (B) Diff-Quik–stained cytology specimen shows loose aggre-gates of atypical epithelial cells with large nuclei, consistent with ductal carcinoma. This proved to be an infiltrating ductal carcinoma at excision. (×160)

use of FNA in clinically or mammographically benign cases resulted in 60 unnecessary biopsies (56 atypia and 4 suspicious) but also detected 33 cancers. The researchers found age to be an independent determinant of the pre-dictive value of FNA. Cancer was found as a result of atypical cytology in 6 of 42 clinically benign cases in women under 40 years of age, compared with 27 of 51 cases in women over 39 years of age, largely due to the tendency of fibroadenomas to have atypical cytology.[45] In addition to fibroadenomas, fibrocystic changes, papil-lomas, and scarring after radiotherapy can rarely be sources of suspicious findings on cytology.[46–48] Phyllodes tumors cannot be reliably differentiated from fibroade-nomas on the basis of cytology.[49]

Lobular carcinomas are particularly challenging both radiologically and cytologically. The diagnostic yield of FNA with lobular carcinomas ranges from 20% to 30%.[41,50] Lobular carcinoma in situ is a particular prob-

lem because it is often an incidental finding on excisional biopsy that is not clearly related to a mammographic abnormality.[51]

Distinguishing tubular carcinoma from radial scar is another challenging area both mammographically and pathologically. Although radial scars tend to be spicu-lated masses with lucent centers mammographically and cancers tend to have dense centers, no reliable distinc-tion can be made. Core needle biopsy and FNA should be avoided in such cases because of the overlap in their appearance microscopically as well.[52]

Distinction of in situ carcinoma from invasive carci-noma is not reliably made on cytologic analysis,[53,54] nor can a determination of invasive cancer be reliably made with core biopsies. In a recent series by Jackman and col-leagues,[55] 19% of histologically invasive cancers were thought to be in situ on analysis of core needle biopsy specimens. As discussed earlier, atypical hyperplasia can

TABLE 2-1. *Histologically correlated fine needle aspirates (cysts excluded)* *

Investigators	N	TP	TN	FP	FN	Susp	Ins	Comments
Franzen & Zajicek, 1960[40,*]	1470	662/873	308/597	1	42	117/140	29/126	17/52 malignant/atypias
Horgan et al, 1991[41]	2000	171/264	1471/1736	3	38	51/58	4/254	—
Gelabert et al, 1990[4]	107	84/95	12/12	0	3	6/6	2/2	—
Arishita et al, 1990[42]	60	13/18	28/42	0	2	—	3/18	Mammographic grid, nonpalpable
Masood et al, 1990[43]	100	17/20	71/80	0	3[†]	—	0/9	Mammographic grid, nonpalpable
Fajardo et al, 1990[44]	100	17/30	54/70	0	7[‡]	6/6	0	Stereotactic guidance, 4/20 malignant/atypias
Ciatto et al, 1989[45,*]	1149	500/1014	NC[§]	2[¶]	NC[§]	372/391	NC[§]	142/288 malignant/atypias
TOTALS	4986	1464/2314	1944/2537	6	95	552/601	38/409	163/360 malignant/atypias

TP, true-positives: cancers called malignant at FNA over total cancers; TN, true-negatives (cases called benign at FNA over total benign lesions); FP, false-positives; FN, false-negatives; Susp, malignancies over cases termed "suspicious" at FNA; Ins, malignancies over cases with "insufficient" samples on FNA.

* Not all patients had excisional biopsies, but the decision to biopsy was independent of the FNA results except for cysts that were excluded from the data presented.

† Two cases of lobular carcinoma in situ and one of ductal carcinoma in situ were considered false-negatives.

‡ Includes two cases of lobular carcinoma in situ adjacent to the mammographic abnormality.

§ Not calculable; a retrospective study of abnormal cytopathology reports.

¶ Two fibroadenomas were interpreted as malignant on FNA.

be similarly problematic both on core needle biopsy and FNA, with many representing in situ or even invasive carcinomas.[55] Analysis of smear pattern has met with variable success, with Layfield and associates[37] showing that an *individual cell predominant* pattern was associated with an increased risk of distant metastases when compared with sheets or cluster-predominant patterns.

Preliminary studies suggest that FNA is less reliable diagnostically for lesions manifested only as microcalcifications,[44,56] but further study is needed. Lofgren and colleagues[56] reported 87% sensitivity and 93% specificity for lesions manifested as microcalcifications, compared with 94% sensitivity and 100% specificity for spiculated tumors and 100% sensitivity *and* specificity for circumscribed masses. This phenomenon has also been observed with core needle biopsy.[57] Indeed, Liberman and associates[58] found that even when additional large-core passes were made through microcalcifications, and when specimen radiography confirmed sampling of the microcalcifications, the sensitivity of the technique resulted in diagnostic material in 87% of cases of microcalcifications after five passes and 92% after six passes, compared with 99% of masses after five passes.

Complications

The greatest risk associated with FNA is the possibility of its being nondiagnostic with the attendant cost and discomfort to the patient. By contrast, large core needle biopsy can be performed for the same cost as FNA and has insufficient sample rates ranging from 3% to 5%,[57] comparable with excisional biopsy. Pneumothorax is a rare complication of FNA, seen in 0.18% of cases in one multicenter review[59]; presumably, it is most likely with lesions close to the chest wall. The risk of pneumothorax can be minimized by infiltrating lidocaine *beneath* the lesion to elevate it from the chest wall and approaching the lesion parallel to the chest wall. Patient discomfort is usually minimal. In rare cases, a clinically detectable hematoma may result. This is most common after radiotherapy, when the vessels are particularly friable. Seeding of the needle track remains a concern. In a series of 29 surgical specimens in which FNA, needle localization, or core biopsy had been performed, Youngson and colleagues[60] found 26 had microscopic evidence of displaced fragments of carcinomatous epithelium in proximity to the area of needle track hemorrhage. Because radiotherapy is usually administered after breast conservation surgery, the clinical significance of such microscopic tumor spread is unknown.

FINE NEEDLE ASPIRATION OF THYROID AND OTHER SUBCUTANEOUS MASSES

Nodular thyroid disease is present in 3% to 8% of adults on physical examination and in up to 30% of adults on imaging studies,[61] with adenomas and goiter representing the bulk of disease. The annual incidence of thyroid cancer is roughly 1 in 25,000 people in the United States. The appropriate management of a thyroid nodule integrates findings on physical examination, clinical history, radionuclide studies, ultrasound, and FNA. A hard, fixed mass on physical examination, obstructive symptoms, adenopathy, or vocal cord paralysis suggests malignancy. Clinical risk factors include age under 25 years (or over 60 years in men), family history, prior irradiation to the neck, and rapid growth of the nodule.

Radionuclide imaging has low specificity but may be

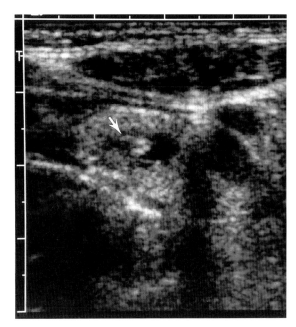

FIG. 2-7. Ultrasound of thyroid adenoma. Ultrasound reveals a predominantly cystic lesion with a small solid hypoechoic component (*arrow*) in this 65-year-old woman with a palpable nodule in the left lobe of the thyroid. Fine needle aspirate was consistent with an adenoma with cystic degeneration.

used as an initial examination to evaluate for an autonomous nodule. Normal thyroid cells trap $^{99m}TcO_4^-$ and trap and organify radioiodine. Most benign and nearly all malignant thyroid nodules show lower concentrations of the radiopharmaceuticals than normal thyroid tissue. Autonomous nodules often have higher concentrations of radiotracer than does normal thyroid, appearing "hot" on radionuclide imaging, and are almost always benign; such nodules can be followed up clinically. If a nodule shows intermediate uptake or appears "cold" relative to normal thyroid, FNA is indicated. Similarly, a dominant nodule in a multinodular goitrous gland should be treated as a solitary nodule, although the risk of malignancy is still lower than for a solitary nodule.

Ultrasonography reveals few simple cysts of the thyroid. Most cystic lesions have hypoechoic mural nodules, and most of these are degenerating adenomas (Fig. 2-7). Cystic lesions larger than 4 cm may require excision, as may lesions that recur after aspiration. Aspiration of such lesions is directed to the solid component but often yields inadequate material because of the bloody nature of the aspirate. Ultrasound is very helpful in guiding FNA of nonpalpable thyroid nodules. Typically, a 25-gauge needle is used in the technique described for breast aspiration. In a Mayo Clinic study of 10,971 FNAs of the thyroid, malignant cells were found in 416 (4%) of aspirates, of which 404 had clinical or tissue diagnosis and malignancy was confirmed in 401 (99%)[62] and 3 (1%) were false-positives. Twelve had no follow-up. Of another 1192 (11%) with suspicious cytologic findings, 984 had tissue diagnosis and, of these, 288

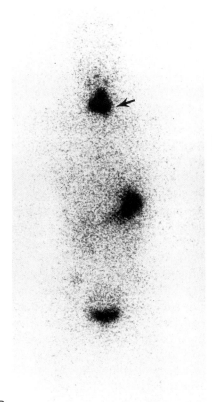

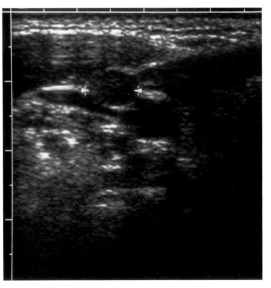

FIG. 2-8. Imaging of recurrent thyroid cancer. **(A)** Anterior ^{131}I whole-body gamma camera image taken 3 months after treatment of papillary thyroid cancer in this 26-year-old woman shows uptake in the thyroid bed (*arrow*). This phenomenon can be normal or reflect residual or recurrent disease. Excretion of radioiodine is also observed in the stomach and bladder. **(B)** Ultrasound revealed a small hypoechoic nodule (*arrowheads*) just anterior to the carotid artery. Ultrasound-guided FNA results revealed recurrent papillary thyroid cancer.

A,B

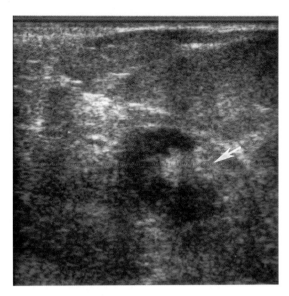

FIG. 2-9. Normal lymph node on ultrasound. Mammography revealed an enlarging, well-defined mass in the axillary portion of the left breast of this 44-year-old woman who had a melanoma of the left arm 4 years earlier. Ultrasound showed the nodule to be well-defined and hypoechoic with an echogenic central fatty hilus (*arrow*), compatible with a lymph node. Ultrasound-guided FNA (and core biopsy) showed normal lymphoid tissue.

tivity and specificity of thyroid FNA range from 71% to 95% and 88% to 100%,[63-65] respectively, and exceed those for pertechnetate scanning and ultrasound.[66]

Radionuclide and ultrasound imaging can be helpful in detecting recurrent disease. Iodine 131 is typically used in whole-body scanning (as well as radiotherapy) in patients with known thyroid cancer. Uptake in the thyroid bed can be normal or can reflect residual or recurrent disease (Fig. 2-8). Metastatic foci usually show significant uptake. Anaplastic thyroid carcinoma, medullary thyroid carcinoma, and some forms of papillary and follicular thyroid carcinoma do not show appreciable uptake of radioiodine.[67]

Other subcutaneous masses, including parathyroid,[68] head and neck tumors,[69] and cutaneous and subcutaneous metastases from internal carcinomas,[70] are readily evaluated by FNA. Ultrasound guidance can be particularly helpful both in directing aspiration of the area of concern and in avoiding adjacent vascular structures.

Detection of nodal disease by imaging methods is unreliable. Many studies describe size and shape criteria for normal lymph nodes, but the specificity of ultrasound, computed tomography, magnetic resonance imaging, and physical examination remain about 60% to 70%.[71,72] Loss of the normal architecture on ultrasound, with loss of the echogenic fatty hilus, can portend malignancy (Figs. 2-9 and 2-10). FNA of lymph nodes has been shown to be 75% to 85% accurate diagnostically.[73,74] The role of large core needle biopsy of nodal disease is not yet fully defined.

(29%) proved malignant. Twenty-one percent of aspirates, 2292, were nondiagnostic or unsatisfactory. There were 18 (0.2% overall) known false-negatives. The sensi-

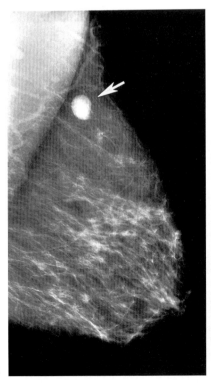

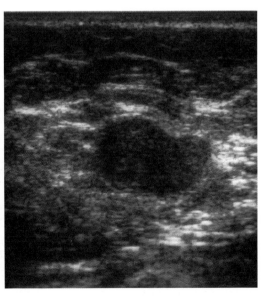

FIG. 2-10. Lymph node with metastatic breast carcinoma. **(A)** In this 60-year-old asymptomatic woman, mediolateral oblique mammogram showed a dramatic increase in the size and density of what had appeared to be a lymph node 2 years earlier (*arrow*). **(B)** Ultrasound was performed, revealing a bean-shaped hypoechoic nodule suggestive of a lymph node, but lacking the normal central echogenic fatty hilus. Ultrasound-guided FNA (as well as core biopsy and excision) showed metastatic infiltrating ductal carcinoma. The primary cancer was not found even at mastectomy.

A,B

CONCLUSIONS

The ideal approach to breast, thyroid, and nodal disease integrates the patient, radiologist, pathologist, and surgeon. Results of physical examination and history, imaging, and biopsy must be correlated to determine optimal patient management. Use of nonsurgical biopsy methods such as FNA and large core needle biopsy requires an understanding of the prebiopsy level of suspicion of disease for reliable interpretation of the pathologic findings. A suspicious lesion with a nonspecific benign or insufficient needle aspirate or core needle biopsy still merits excisional biopsy.

REFERENCES

1. Baker LH. Breast Cancer Detection Demonstration Project: five year summary report. CA 1982;32:194.
2. Ciatto S, Cataliotti L, Distante V. Nonpalpable lesions detected with mammography: review of 512 consecutive cases. Radiology 1987;165:99.
3. Tabar L, Gad A. Screening for breast cancer: the Swedish trial. Radiology 1981;138:219.
4. Gelabert HA, Hsiu JG, Mullen JT, et al. Prospective evaluation of the role of fine-needle aspiration biopsy in the diagnosis and management of patients with palpable solid breast lesions. Am Surg 1990;56:263.
5. Lindfors KK, Rosenquist CJ. Needle core biopsy guided with mammography: a study of cost-effectiveness. Radiology 1994;190:217.
6. Liberman L, Fahs MC, Dershaw DD, et al. Impact of stereotaxic core breast biopsy on cost of diagnosis. Radiology 1995;195:633.
7. Rubin E, Dempsey PJ, Pile NS, et al. Needle-localization biopsy of the breast: impact of a selective core needle biopsy program on yield. Radiology 1995;195:627.
8. Holland R, Veling S, Mravunac M, et al. Histologic multifocality of Tis, T1-2 breast carcinomas. Cancer 1985;56:979.
9. Edeiken S. Mammography and palpable cancer of the breast. Cancer 1988;61:263.
10. Brenner RJ, Bein ME, Sarti DA, et al. Spontaneous regression of interval benign cysts of the breast. Radiology 1994;193:365.
11. Fajardo LL, Jackson VP, Hunter TB. Interventional procedures in diseases of the breast: needle biopsy, pneumocystography, and galactography. AJR 1992;158:1231.
12. Fornage BD. Percutaneous biopsies of the breast: state of the art. (Review) Cardiovasc Intervent Radiol 1991;14:29.
13. Ikeda DM, Helvie MA, Adler DD, et al. The role of fine-needle aspiration and pneumocystography in the treatment of impalpable breast cysts. AJR 1992;158:1239.
14. Ciatto S, Cariaggi P, Bulgaresi P. The value of routine cytologic examination of breast cyst fluids. Acta Cytol 1987;31:301.
15. Sickles EA. Periodic mammographic follow-up of probably benign lesions: results in 3184 consecutive cases. Radiology 1991;179:463.
16. Sickles EA. Nonpalpable, circumscribed, noncalcified solid breast masses: likelihood of malignancy based on lesion size and age of patient. Radiology 1994;192:439.
17. Logan-Young WW, Hoffman NY, Janus JA. Fine-needle aspiration cytology in the detection of breast cancer in nonsuspicious lesions. Radiology 1992;184:49.
18. Franquet T, Cozolluela R, DeMiguel C. Stereotaxic fine-needle aspiration of low-suspicion, nonpalpable breast nodules: valid alternative to follow-up mammography. Radiology 1992;183:635.
19. Malberger E, Edoute Y, Toledano O, et al. Fine-needle aspiration and cytologic findings of surgical scar lesions in women with breast cancer. Cancer 1992;69:148.
20. Palombini L, Fulciniti F, Vetrani A, et al. Fine-needle aspiration biopsies of breast masses: a critical analysis of 1956 cases in 8 years (1976–1984). Cancer 1988;61:2273.
21. Zarbo RJ, Howanitz PJ, Bachner P. Interinstitutional comparison of performance in breast fine-needle aspiration cytology. Arch Pathol Lab Med 1991;115:743.
22. Evans WP, Cade SH. Needle localization and fine-needle aspiration biopsy of nonpalpable breast lesions with use of standard and stereotactic equipment. Radiology 1989;173:53.
23. Helvie MA, Baker DE, Adler DD, et al. Radiographically guided fine-needle aspiration of nonpalpable breast lesions. Radiology 1990;174:657.
24. Gordon PB, Goldenberg SL, Chan NHL. Solid breast lesions: diagnosis with US-guided fine-needle aspiration biopsy. Radiology 1993;189:573.
25. Fornage BD, Coan JD, David CL. Ultrasound-guided needle biopsy of the breast and other interventional procedures. (Review) Radiol Clin North Am 1992;30:167.
26. Ciatto S, Catarzi S, Morrone D, et al. Fine-needle aspiration cytology of nonpalpable breast lesions: US versus stereotactic guidance. Radiology 1993;188:195.
27. Patel JJ, Gartell PC, Smallwood JA, et al. Fine needle aspiration cytology of breast masses: an evaluation of its accuracy and reasons for diagnostic failure. Ann R Coll Surg Engl 1987;69:156.
28. Pennes DR, Naylor B, Rebner M. Fine needle aspiration biopsy of the breast: influence of the number of passes and the sample size on the diagnostic yield. Acta Cytol 1990;34:673.
29. Akhtar M, Ali MA, Huq M, et al. Fine-needle biopsy: comparison of cellular yield with and without aspiration. Diagn Cytopathol 1989;5:162.
30. Mair S, Dunbar F, Becker PJ, et al. Fine needle cytology—is aspiration suction necessary? A study of 100 masses in various sites. Acta Cytol 1989;33:809.
31. Frable WJ. Needle aspiration of the breast. Cancer 1984;53:671.
32. Wilkinson EJ, Bland KI. Techniques and results of aspiration cytology for diagnosis of benign and malignant diseases of the breast. Surg Clin North Am 1990;70:801.
33. Masood S. Fluorescent cytochemical detection of estrogen and progesterone receptors in breast fine-needle aspirates. Am J Clin Pathol 1991;95:35.
34. Kitchen PRB, Stillwell RG, Henderson MA, et al. Oestrogen receptor assay of breast cancer by immunocytochemistry of fine needle aspirates. Aust N Z J Surg 1991;61:223.
35. Nizzoli R, Bozzetti C, Savoldi L, et al. Immunocytochemical assay of estrogen and progesterone receptors in fine needle aspirates from breast cancer patients. Acta Cytol 1994;38:933.
36. Remvikos Y, Magdelenat H, Zajdela A. DNA flow cytometry applied to fine needle sampling of human breast cancer. Cancer 1988;61:1629.
37. Layfield LJ, Robert ME, Cramer H, et al. Aspiration biopsy smear pattern as a predictor of biologic behavior in adenocarcinoma of the breast. Acta Cytol 1992;36:208.
38. Giard R, Hermans J. The value of aspiration cytologic examination of the breast: a statistical review of the medical literature. Cancer 1992;69:2104.
39. Jackson VP. The status of mammographically guided fine needle aspiration biopsy of nonpalpable breast lesions. (Review) Radiol Clin North Am 1992;30:155.
40. Franzen S, Zajicek J. Aspiration biopsy in the diagnosis of palpable lesions of the breast: critical review of 3479 consecutive biopsies. Acta Radiol 1960;7:241.
41. Horgan PG, Waldron D, Mooney E, et al. The role of aspiration cytologic examination in the diagnosis of carcinoma of the breast. Surg Gynecol Obstet 1991;172:290.
42. Arishita GI, Cruz BK, Harding CT, et al. Mammogram-directed fine-needle aspiration of nonpalpable breast lesions. J Surg Oncol 1991;48:153.
43. Masood S, Frykberg ER, McLellan GL, et al. Prospective evaluation of radiologically directed fine-needle aspiration biopsy of nonpalpable breast lesions. Cancer 1990;66:1480.
44. Fajardo LL, Davis JR, Wiens JL, et al. Mammography-guided stereotactic fine-needle aspiration cytology of nonpalpable breast lesions: prospective comparison with surgical biopsy results. AJR 1990;155:977.

45. Ciatto S, Cecchini S, Grazzini G, et al. Positive predictive value of fine needle aspiration cytology of breast lesions. Acta Cytol 1989; 33:894.

46. Mulford DK, Dawson AE. Atypia in fine needle aspiration cytology of nonpalpable and palpable mammographically detected breast lesions. Acta Cytol 1994;38:9.

47. Al-Kaisi N. The spectrum of the "gray zone" in breast cytology: a review of 186 cases of atypical and suspicious cytology. Acta Cytol 1994;38:898.

48. Gupta RK. Radiation-induced cellular changes in the breast: a potential diagnostic pitfall in fine needle aspiration cytology. Acta Cytol 1989;33:141.

49. Shimizu K, Masawa N, Yamada T, et al. Cytologic evaluation of phyllodes tumors as compared to fibroadenomas of the breast. Acta Cytol 1994;38:891.

50. Hajdu SI, Gaston JP. Aspiration cytology of breast. (Review) Clin Lab Med 1991;11:357.

51. Sonnenfeld MR, Frenna TH, Weidner N, et al. Lobular carcinoma in situ: mammographic-pathologic correlation of results of needle-directed biopsy. Radiology 1991;181:363.

52. DeLaTorre M, Lindholm K, Lindgren A. Fine needle aspiration cytology of tubular breast carcinoma and radial scar. Acta Cytol 1994;38:884.

53. Venegas R, Rutgers JL, Cameron BL, et al. Fine needle aspiration cytology of breast ductal carcinoma in situ. Acta Cytol 1994;38:136.

54. Sneige N, White VA, Katz RL, et al. Ductal carcinoma-in-situ of the breast: fine-needle aspiration cytology of 12 cases. Diagn Cytopathol 1989;5:371.

55. Jackman RJ, Nowels KW, Shepard MJ, et al. Stereotaxic large-core needle biopsy of 450 nonpalpable breast lesions with surgical correlation in lesions with cancer or atypical hyperplasia. Radiology 1994;193:91.

56. Lofgren M, Andersson I, Lindhom K. Stereotactic fine-needle aspiration for cytologic diagnosis of nonpalpable breast lesions. AJR 1990;154:1191.

57. Parker SH, Burbank F, Jackman RJ, et al. Percutaneous large-core breast biopsy: a multi-institutional study. Radiology 1994;193:359.

58. Liberman L, Dershaw DD, Rosen PP, et al. Stereotaxic 14-gauge breast biopsy: how many core biopsy specimens are needed? Radiology 1994;192:793.

59. Catania S, Boccato P, Bono A, et al. Pneumothorax: a rare complication of fine needle aspiration of the breast. Acta Cytol 1989;33:140.

60. Youngson B, Cranor M, Rosen PP. Epithelial displacement in surgical breast specimens following needling procedures. Am J Surg Pathol 1994;18:896.

61. Hay ID, Klee GG. Thyroid cancer diagnosis and management. Clin Lab Med 1993;13:725.

62. Gharib H, Goellner J, Johnson D. Fine-needle aspiration biopsy of the thyroid: a 12-year experience with 11,000 biopsies. Clin Lab Med 1993;13:699.

63. Gharib H. Fine-needle aspiration biopsy of thyroid nodules: advantages, limitations, and effect. (Review) Mayo Clin Proc 1994;69:44.

64. Altavilla G, Pascale M, Nenci I. Fine needle aspiration cytology of thyroid gland diseases. Acta Cytol 1990;34:251.

65. Atkinson BF. Fine needle aspiration of the thyroid. (Review) Monogr Pathol 1993;1993:166.

66. Jones A, Aitman TJ, Edmonds CJ, et al. Comparison of fine needle aspiration cytology, radioisotopic and ultrasound scanning in the management of thyroid nodules. Postgrad Med J 1990;66:914.

67. Reading CC, Gorman CA. Thyroid imaging techniques. (Review) Clin Lab Med 1993;13:711.

68. Shapiro MJ, Batang ES. Needle aspiration biopsy of the thyroid and parathyroid. (Review) Otolaryngol Clin North Am 1990;23:217.

69. Flynn MB, Wolfson SE, Thomas S, et al. Fine needle aspiration biopsy in clinical management of head and neck tumors. J Surg Oncol 1990;44:214.

70. Srinivasan R, Ray R, Nijhawan R. Metastatic cutaneous and subcutaneous deposits from internal carcinoma. An analysis of cases diagnosed by fine needle aspiration. Acta Cytol 1993;37:894.

71. Pamilo M, Soiva M, Lavast E. Real-time ultrasound, axillary mammography, and clinical examination in the detection of axillary lymph node metastases in breast cancer patients. J Ultr Med 1989;8:115.

72. March DE, Wechsler RJ, Kurtz AB, et al. CT-Pathologic correlation of axillary lymph nodes in breast carcinoma. J Comput Assist Tomogr 1991;15:440.

73. Royston D. Fine needle aspiration biopsy of lymph nodes and subcutaneous masses. Ir J Med Sci 1993;162:21.

74. Frable WJ, Kardos TF. Fine needle aspiration biopsy: applications in the diagnosis of lymphoproliferative diseases. Am J Surg Pathol 1988;12(Suppl 1):6.

Fine Needle Aspiration of Subcutaneous Organs and Masses,
edited by Yener S. Erozan and Thomas A. Bonfiglio.
Lippincott–Raven Publishers, Philadelphia, © 1996.

CHAPTER 3

Fine Needle Aspiration of the Breast

Andrea E. Dawson

The incidence of breast carcinoma in the United States has increased to its current alarming rate of one in eight women. Although 5-year survival rates have not changed significantly during the past 25 years, it is clear that women with small localized breast tumors and negative lymph nodes have the best prognosis.[1-3] Consequently, early detection of breast cancer has assumed increasing importance as a means of improving the survival from this deadly disease. Although physical examination and self-examination are essential in the detection of breast masses, widespread mammographic screening has had a more significant impact in the detection of smaller and earlier breast lesions.[2] However, mammographic screening alone has a sensitivity of about 80%, whereas its specificity is only 15% to 25%.[4-7] Fine needle aspiration (FNA) is one way to improve the specificity of mammography without resorting to open surgical biopsy for all of the lesions that are detected. FNA has proved to be a valuable relatively noninvasive procedure for evaluating palpable and mammographically detected nonpalpable lesions. It was initially developed by Martin, Ellis, and Stewart in 1930.[8,9] Its initial acceptance was in Scandinavia, where it has been widely used for many years. The acceptance in the United States has been slower, but in recent years it has become a widely practiced diagnostic procedure with excellent reported sensitivity and specificity rates.[10-16] Although most of these data are based on aspiration of palpable breast masses, aspiration of nonpalpable lesions has also been shown to be an effective diagnostic procedure.[17-20] FNA has several advantages over the traditional open surgical biopsy. It is a diagnostic procedure that can be performed in any office or mammography clinic.[21] A rapid, cost-effective diagnosis can be provided to reassure the anxious patient or allow development of a therapeutic plan if a diagnosis of malignancy is rendered.[22] A diagnosis of malignancy by FNA enables the patient to proceed to either lumpectomy and axillary node dissection or mastectomy without an additional open excisional biopsy.[15,21]

Of the several criticisms of breast FNA, false-negative diagnosis is most often cited as a weakness of the technique. False-negative rates vary among series, ranging from 0.7% to 22%.[23,24] To improve the diagnostic reliability of the procedure, some researchers have recom-

A. E. Dawson: Department of Pathology and Laboratory Medicine, University of Rochester Medical Center, Rochester, NY 14642.

mended that the findings on physical examination, mammography, and FNA (ie, Triple-Test) be taken into account before a diagnosis is rendered.[25] Close communication among the physicians involved in the diagnosis and care of the patient is essential to avoid both false-negative and false-positive diagnoses. Other factors that contribute to the accuracy of the diagnosis include the proficiency of the aspirator, experience of the pathologist, and the palpability and size of the lesion. In addition, special histologic subtypes of cancer, such as tubular and mucinous carcinomas, may contribute to false-negative diagnoses in FNA of the breast because of their low-grade cytologic features.[23,26] The false-positive diagnostic rate in the literature is much lower than the false-negative rate. A false-positive diagnosis is considered unacceptable, however, because a mastectomy or lumpectomy with axillary node dissection may be performed on the basis of the FNA diagnosis alone in many institutions.

This chapter begins with a discussion of the technical aspects that are important to FNA and a general approach to FNA of the breast for both palpable and nonpalpable lesions. In addition, a wide range of benign and malignant lesions that may be encountered in any FNA practice are described with attention to the cytologic features and the pitfalls in diagnosis. Breast cytology can be difficult because of the many gray or borderline areas, such as the diagnosis of proliferative breast disease, carcinoma in situ, papillary neoplasms, and low-grade cancers. In these borderline diagnostic areas, the focus is on providing diagnostic clues and formulating an approach that may be helpful in suggesting the correct diagnosis. Finally, technologies such as flow cytometry, nuclear grading, and immunocytochemical methods are briefly discussed as potential ways of providing the maximum

amount of diagnostic, prognostic, and therapeutic information from the breast FNA.

TECHNICAL ASPECTS

General

Aspiration can be performed on both palpable and nonpalpable lesions.[27] Nonpalpable lesions require imaging techniques such as ultrasound and mammographic and stereotactic methods to aid in localization of the lesion[28–31] (see Chap. 2). For most aspirates, a 22- to 23-gauge, 1.5-inch needle is used; it is attached to a 20-mL syringe fitted in a commercially available holder (see Chap. 1). The number of passes that are performed varies with the nature of the lesion and the experience of the operator. Some reports recommend three or four aspirations per lesion,[32] but most aspirates we receive are from one aspirate with good results.[19] Smears are either fixed immediately in 95% ethyl alcohol for Papanicolaou stain or air-dried and stained by a modified rapid Wright (Diff-Quik) stain.[10] In many practices, air-dried Diff-Quik–stained slides are assessed immediately for adequacy. If the specimen is insufficient, more passes are performed to obtain adequate material. This triage approach can allow for additional passes for special studies such as flow cytometry or tumor marker studies.[33] In our practice, most smears are obtained in an outpatient mammography clinic. FNA smears are rapidly fixed in 95% ethyl alcohol and then sent to cytopathology for staining and interpretation. To obtain optimal results with the Papanicolaou stain, the slides must be fixed rapidly in alcohol to avoid drying artifact. Drying enlarges the nuclei and can be the cause of a false-positive or false-suspicious diagnosis (Fig. 3-1).

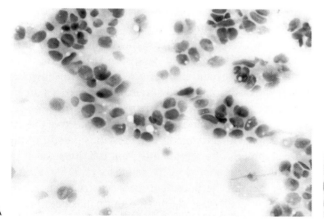
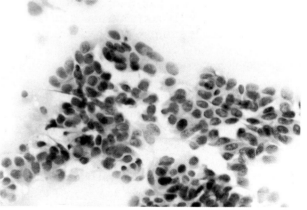

A

B

FIG. 3-1. Drying artifact. **(A)** This aspirate illustrates the pitfall of drying artifact. The aspirate was diagnosed as suggestive of carcinoma due to increased cellularity, single epithelial cells, and artifactually enlarged nuclei (secondary to drying). The biopsy diagnosis was fibrocystic changes. (Papanicolaou stain, ×100) **(B)** This aspirate has features similar to those shown in **A**, but here the biopsy was diagnostic of infiltrating carcinoma. The similarity between the two aspirates shows the potential for a false-positive diagnosis when marked drying artifact is present. (Papanicolaou stain, ×100)

Stereotactic Localization

The detection of occult breast cancers has increased dramatically with the widespread use of screening mammography.[2,7] In the past, an open biopsy was performed on most mammographically detected lesions but only 10% to 20% of such biopsies were cancerous.[34] A stereotactic technique for evaluation of occult breast lesions was initially developed by Bolmgren and later evaluated by Nordenstrom.[35] A stereotactic device compresses the breast and localizes the exact site of the lesion (microcalcifications, soft shadows, or both) by means of a coordinate system (see Chap. 2). The breast lesions can be localized and sampled with FNA to within 1 mm. The procedure can be performed with minimal patient discomfort and complications.[18,28,29] The stereotactic localization takes more time than FNA performed on palpable lesions but still requires only about 30 minutes. Several studies have compared the result of stereotactic FNA with the subsequent open biopsy result. In these studies, the sensitivity and specificity of the stereotactic FNA is excellent, ranging from 93% to 97%.[28,29] In up to 20% of cases, it is difficult to obtain representative cytologic material (insufficient aspirates) because of several factors, including technical aspects inherent in the stereotactic method, extensive fibrosis in the lesion, minimal disease, a mobile lesion, or a combination of these factors.[27–29,36,37]

In some institutions, stereotactic FNA and stereotactic core needle biopsy are performed on every noncystic lesion to improve the diagnostic yield.[36,37] Stereotactic core needle biopsy uses a 14-gauge needle with several cores of tissue removed for processing and diagnosis in surgical pathology.[36–42] Some reports comparing stereotactic FNA and stereotactic core needle biopsy have found that stereotactic FNA is better at diagnosing malignant microcalcifications, presumably because of increased sampling of the area of interest. Stereotactic core needle biopsy may be better suited for diagnosing other types of lesions. The guidelines for appropriate use of stereotactic FNA and stereotactic core needle biopsy are undergoing clinical evaluation. The use of more precise localizing techniques in conjunction with FNA is improving the specificity of mammography and decreasing the need for open surgical biopsies. Even with these improved technologies and diagnostic procedures, however, it is essential to take into account the cytologic, clinical, and mammographic findings to determine the appropriate plan for patient management.

DIAGNOSTIC ASPECTS

Approach to Cytopathologic Diagnosis

The successful use of FNA for evaluation of breast lesions requires cooperation and a team approach among the clinicians involved in the patient's care. This is true for both palpable and nonpalpable mammographically detected breast lesions. It is critical to take into account the clinical mammographic impressions and the FNA diagnosis. If these do not correlate, communication between physicians is essential.[15,21,33] Diagnoses can be stratified based on the cytologic features into the following categories: definite for malignancy, probable or suggestive of malignancy, and benign condition or negative for malignancy. These diagnoses often can be derived from the cytology alone; if the clinical picture is incorporated, however, a greater degree of diagnostic certainty results.[43] If a negative diagnosis is made and the clinical or mammographic findings or both are suggestive, these patients should proceed to biopsy (Fig. 3-2).

The initial evaluation of the FNA smear should be performed on low power. A low-power scan of the slides provides information about the cellularity, the overall pattern, and the adequacy of the aspirate. The criteria for malignancy rely, in general, on cellularity, atypia, and epithelial discohesion (Table 3-1). Cellularity plays an important role in the diagnosis of breast malignancy and can be assessed quickly on a low-power scan. In fine needle aspirates from the breast, the pattern or architecture also has a critical role in diagnosis. For example, the biphasic pattern of staghorn fronds and the background naked nuclei that are seen in a fibroadenoma are best appreciated on low power (Fig. 3-3). After the evaluation of the low-power characteristics, individual cells and groups of epithelial cells should be evaluated under high power to provide information such as degree of nuclear atypia, cellular overlap, and the nature of the single epithelial cells and background cells (Fig. 3-4). In most breast fine needle aspirates that are evaluated using this approach, the cytopathologist can arrive at a accurate malignant or benign diagnosis (Table 3-1).

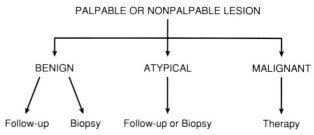

FIG. 3-2. Management of breast lesion evaluated by FNA. This diagram illustrates the general management of either a nonpalpable or a palpable breast lesion. If the clinical or radiographic impression is benign and there is a benign FNA diagnosis, the patient can be followed clinically. If the impression is suspicious and the FNA diagnosis is benign, the patient must have further work-up consisting of repeat FNA, core biopsy, or open biopsy. Any atypical diagnosis warrants further diagnostic work-up, although in certain situations the patient can have close follow-up. A malignant FNA diagnosis can be followed up by definitive therapy in the appropriate clinical setting.

TABLE 3-1. *General cytologic features: benign versus malignant*

Cytologic feature	Benign	Malignant
Cellularity	Low	Moderate to high
Epithelial groups	Honeycomb	Overlapping, three-dimensional clusters
Single epithelial cells	Rare	Numerous
Nuclear atypia	Minimal	Minimal to marked
Diathesis	Absent	Can be present

Negative Diagnosis

A diagnosis of negative is nonspecific and is used when there is no evidence of malignancy and when specific diagnostic features of a benign lesion are not present. When FNA is performed on women with nonpalpable mammographic lesions with low clinical suspicion for malignancy, a significant percentage of these aspirates are from normal breast tissue. These aspirates have low cellularity with scattered fragments of adipose tissue and benign epithelial cell clusters. In this patient population there may be only three or four epithelial clusters per aspirate (Fig. 3-5). Apocrine metaplastic and foam cells may also be present. Although guidelines for adequacy are not well established for a fine needle aspirate from a low suspicious lesion, an adequate smear requires that at least three adipose tissue groups or epithelial groups are present on the slide. The general guidelines for adequacy when FNA is performed on a palpable mass require increased cellularity, depending on the clinical situation.

Atypical or Suspicious Diagnoses

Although FNA plays an important role in the evaluation of breast lesions in conjunction with mammo-graphic screening, the aspiration of early or small lesions may lead to increased atypical or suspicious cytologic diagnoses.[44] Increased atypical diagnoses may decrease the excellent reported sensitivity and specificity of breast FNA, which will result in an unacceptable rate of open surgical biopsies for benign lesions. In this era of cost containment, one role of FNA is to reassure both the patient and the clinician that a breast lesion is benign, alleviating the need for the more expensive open surgical biopsy. Equivocal diagnoses can be due to several factors, including (1) technical factors, in which smears are obscured by blood or drying artifact; (2) inexperience in cytopathologic interpretation; and (3) overlap between benign and malignant features.[45] The atypical diagnosis can be used in the following contexts: the cytopathologist thinks that the cytologic findings in aspirate have met many but not all the criteria for the diagnosis of malignancy, and the FNA specimen has features that are worrisome and deserve close follow-up or further diagnostic testing. In the atypical or suspicious diagnostic category, further diagnostic studies such as either open excisional biopsy or the more recently developed stereotactic core biopsy[41,42] should be performed to confirm a diagnosis of malignancy before proceeding to definitive therapy. Patients with an atypical diagnosis may or may not have lesions that are suggestive of malignancy. In this subset

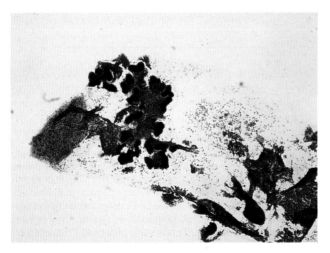

FIG. 3-3. Fibroadenoma. The diagnostic cytologic pattern of a fibroadenoma is present in this low-power photomicrograph. This pattern includes staghorn epithelial groups, stroma, and bipolar cells. (Papanicolaou stain, ×20)

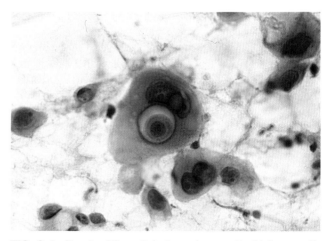

FIG. 3-4. Poorly differentiated carcinoma. On high magnification, markedly pleomorphic single epithelial cells are easily diagnosed as malignant. (Papanicolaou stain, ×300)

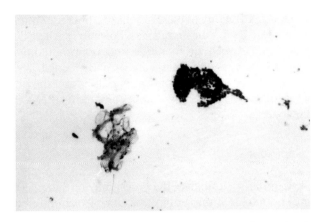

FIG. 3-5. Negative aspirate. A typical aspirate from a benign nonpalpable or small lesion may consist of only scattered clusters of benign epithelial cells and adipose tissue. (Papanicolaou stain, ×50)

of patients, clinical correlation is essential and further diagnostic work-up is often necessary. Several groups have reported their experience with the atypical breast FNA diagnoses.[44-47] Stanley and colleagues[46] showed that atypical diagnoses could be secondary to a variety of pathologic lesions and were not necessarily indicative of atypical proliferative lesions. Al-Kaisi[45] reported that fibroadenomas constituted the largest single cause of an equivocal diagnosis in a review of atypical diagnoses after technical factors and errors due to inexperience were excluded. It has been well documented that there is overlap between the features of fibroadenoma, fibrocystic change, and well-differentiated carcinomas.[47,48] Some investigators have suggested that image analysis can even aid in the correct identification of these overlapping features.[4] At our institution, the incidence of atypical diagnoses in 1990 to 1991 was 5.8% (220 of 3789 aspirates).[44] The biopsy follow-up in these cases was reviewed, and our findings were similar to those reported by others.[45,47] In the atypical suspicious category, there were 86 cases: 10 benign diagnoses and 76 malignancy diagnoses. Biopsy diagnoses in the 10 benign cases included three fibroadenomas, three fibrocystic changes, three papillomas, and one scar after radiation. In the atypical diagnostic category, there were 134 cases with 72 benign and 62 malignant open biopsy diagnoses. Common benign diagnoses in the atypical category included fibroadenoma and fibrocystic changes (46%). Cytologic features responsible for an atypical diagnosis in confirmed benign cases included increased cellularity, single epithelial cells, and reactive nuclear atypia. Our study concluded that an atypical diagnosis rate of less 5% could be achieved by close attention to (1) reactive atypia in the setting of fibrocystic change and fibroadenoma, (2) significance of atypia in an inflammatory smear, and (3) improved sampling and sample preparation. Peterse and colleagues reported that features in favor of benignancy

were monolayers, smooth nuclear borders, and bipolar (naked) nuclei.[47] Features of malignancy were cell dissociation, irregular nuclear borders, and nucleoli. By applying these features retrospectively, the researchers were able to increase diagnostic specificity and sensitivity. If FNA is to be effective at alleviating the necessity for open surgical biopsy, a low incidence of atypical diagnoses must be rendered by careful cytologic interpretation and correlation with clinical and mammographic findings.

CYST ASPIRATION

Aspiration of benign cysts can be therapeutic as well as diagnostic. Because carcinoma is rarely associated with cysts, the value of examining all cyst fluid is controversial.[50,51] In most cytopathology laboratories, cyst fluids are not routinely sent for evaluation. However, proper evaluation of cyst fluid is indicated in two settings: when the cyst fluid is bloody and when the cyst only partially collapses after FNA. In both instances, the incidence of malignancy is increased.[51] Clear or light yellow cyst fluid is almost always paucicellular. The cellularity consists of foam cells and variable numbers of apocrine metaplastic and benign ductal cells (Fig. 3-6).

CYTOLOGIC FINDINGS IN CYST FLUIDS
- Many foam cells (histiocytes)
- Apocrine metaplastic cells
- Benign ductal cells
- Scattered chronic inflammatory cells

Benign apocrine metaplastic cells in a cyst fluid may have atypical nuclear features, such as prominent macronucleoli (Fig. 3-7). These apocrine cells may be interpreted as atypical and lead to a false-suspicious diagnosis. If a cyst aspirate has low cellularity and atypical apocrine metaplastic cells or ductal cells, the clinical in-

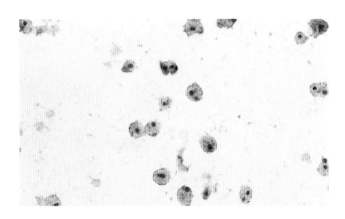

FIG. 3-6. Cyst aspirate. The typical appearance of benign cyst fluid, which contains numerous histiocytes with hemosiderin-laden macrophages. (Papanicolaou stain, ×200)

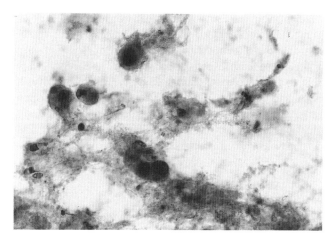

FIG. 3-7. Cyst aspirate—apocrine metaplasia. In benign cysts, apocrine metaplastic cells can have atypical features including enlarged nuclei and nucleoli. The clinical information that the cyst has completely collapsed after aspiration can be helpful in preventing a false-positive diagnosis. (Papanicolaou stain, ×200)

formation that the cyst has completely collapsed is helpful in preventing overdiagnosis. The diagnosis of a malignancy in a cyst fluid relies on the same criteria as does that for a mass lesion, including increased cellularity, single epithelial cells, and nuclear atypia (Fig. 3-8).

BENIGN LESIONS

Fine needle aspiration has been accepted for its role in diagnosing malignancy.[11-13] It is also useful for providing definitive benign diagnosis such as fibroadenoma, fibrocystic changes, and inflammatory lesions.[52,53] Criteria for the diagnosis of many of these lesions (eg, fibroadenoma) are well described.[48] In some areas, however, such as the distinction between proliferative and nonproliferative fibrocystic changes, the criteria are less well defined. This section describes a variety of benign lesions and the pitfalls in diagnosis that may be encountered in FNA of these lesions.

Inflammation

Inflammatory lesions of the breast may mimic malignancy both on mammography and clinical examination. Inflammatory lesions of the breast may be accompanied by marked reactive atypia (Fig. 3-9), which can lead to a false-positive diagnosis of cancer. When an acute or mixed inflammatory infiltrate is present, caution should be exercised before making a diagnosis of malignancy.[44,54]

Mastitis

Acute suppurative mastitis usually occurs in the early post-partum period. *Staphylococcus* organisms, followed by *Streptococcus* species, are the most common etiologic agents.[54a] Aspirates have sheets of neutrophils with scattered reactive epithelial cells (Fig. 3-10). Other types of mastitis include chronic mastitis, plasma cell mastitis, and granulomatous mastitis. Granulomatous mastitis has foreign-body giant cells and a chronic inflammatory infiltrate on the fine needle aspirates.

Fat Necrosis

Fat necrosis is another condition known to mimic cancer on clinical examination and mammography. It often

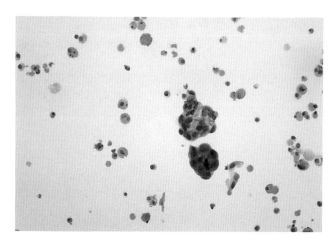

FIG. 3-8. Malignancy in a cyst. Clusters of malignant cells are present in this aspirate, which contains numerous background histiocytes that suggest origin from a cyst. This aspirate was sent for evaluation because a residual mass was present after cyst aspiration. (Papanicolaou stain, ×100)

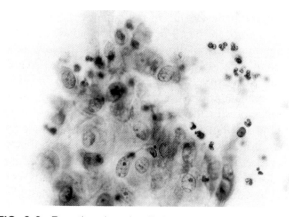

FIG. 3-9. Reactive ductal cells in mastitis. Ductal epithelial cells with reactive features, which include nuclear enlargement and nucleoli in the setting of acute inflammation, are a pitfall for the diagnosis of malignancy. This aspirate was from a case of acute mastitis. (Papanicolaou stain, ×200)

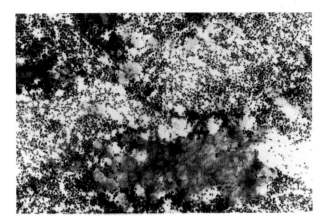

FIG. 3-10. Acute mastitis. Sheets of neutrophils and fibrin are present in this aspirate of acute mastitis. (Papanicolaou stain, ×100)

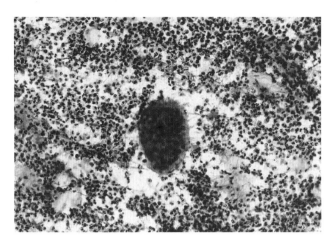

FIG. 3-12. Keratin cyst. Foreign-body giant cells, acute inflammation, and keratinous debris are present in this aspirate of a keratin cyst. (Papanicolaou stain, ×100)

occurs following trauma or foreign-body reaction or in response to malignancy. A history of prior trauma may or may not be given by the patient.[55] The FNA findings of fat necrosis consist of fat, debris, inflammatory cells, and lipid-laden macrophages (Fig. 3-11).

CYTOLOGIC FINDINGS IN FAT NECROSIS
- Lipid-laden macrophages
- Acute and chronic inflammation
- Epithelial cells admixed in adipose tissue

Aspiration of a ruptured keratin cyst reveals a similar picture, with the addition of keratinous debris and numerous squamous cells in the background (Fig. 3-12).

Subareolar Abscess

Subareolar abscess is a distinct clinical and pathologic entity in which abscess formation is followed by cycles of sinus tract drainage, healing, and recurrence in the subareolar region.[56] Squamous metaplasia of the lactiferous

sinuses is seen by histologic examination, and some believe that this is important in the pathogenesis of this entity. Because nipple retraction may be present, subareolar abscess may be clinically confused with a malignancy. A spectrum of cytologic features have been appreciated by FNA, including anucleated squamous cells, neutrophils, strips of squamous epithelium, and foreign-body giant cells (Fig. 3-13).[57]

CYTOLOGIC FINDINGS OF SUBAREOLAR ABSCESS
- Anucleated squamous cells, squamous epithelium
- Acute and chronic inflammation
- Foreign-body giant cells
- Ductal epithelial atypia.

Many of the findings in subareolar abscess demonstrate diagnostic pitfalls for a false-positive diagnosis. These include atypical ductal cells, atypical squamous cells, and fragments of granulation tissue. The constella-

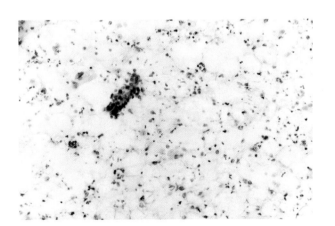

FIG. 3-11. Fat necrosis. This FNA of fat necrosis consists of adipose tissue with numerous histiocytes, inflammation, and occasional ductal epithelial cells. (Papanicolaou stain, ×100)

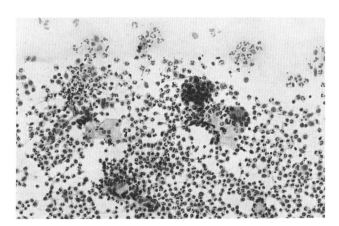

FIG. 3-13. Subareolar abscess. Numerous acute and chronic inflammatory cells with keratinous debris and giant cells are present. (Papanicolaou stain, ×200)

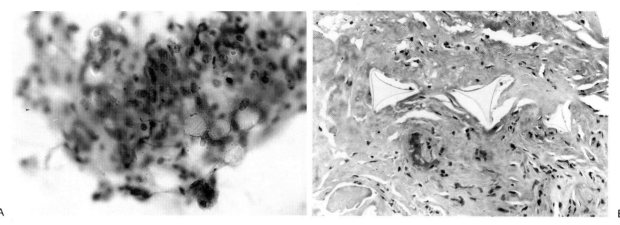

A

B

FIG. 3-14. Fine needle aspirate of silicone rupture. **(A)** The aspirate comprises numerous foreign-body giant cells with engulfed fragments of a silicone capsule implant. (Papanicolaou stain, ×200) **(B)** The biopsy specimen from the same patient shows refractile capsular material in fibrotic tissue consistent with a ruptured silicone implant. (Hematoxylin–eosin stain, ×200)

tion of clinical and cytopathologic findings in the appropriate location should enable the cytopathologist to suggest the diagnosis. The findings may be similar to aspiration of a ruptured epidermal inclusion cyst. The location is helpful in sorting out the differential diagnosis because epidermal cysts are usually peripherally located. Recognition of this lesion is important, because it has a tendency to recur and should be surgically excised.[56]

Other Inflammatory Changes

Women with silicone breast implants may present with firm areas that may be worrisome for malignancy, particularly in patients with a history of breast cancer. FNA is ideally suited for evaluating these lesions. The differential diagnosis in this setting includes: scar tissue, malignancy and reaction to a ruptured silicone implant.

The cytologic findings of a ruptured silicone implant include low to moderate cellularity with numerous histiocytes, chronic inflammatory cells, and foreign-body giant cells. The histiocytes and foreign-body giant cells may contain refractile clear material consistent with capsular polyurethane (Fig. 3-14).[58]

Reparative and reactive lesions such as nodular fasciitis may mimic cancer clinically and mammographically and can be sampled by FNA. Nodular fasciitis is a rapidly growing fibroblastic proliferation resembling granulation tissue. The cytologic findings show cohesive clusters and single spindle cells with variable cellular fragments of collagenous stroma and plump, ganglion-like cells (Fig. 3-15).[59] The clinical history of rapid growth is important, because the differential diagnosis is broad, including spindle cell neoplasms such as fibromatosis, phyllodes tumor, and low-grade metaplastic carcinoma.[60,61]

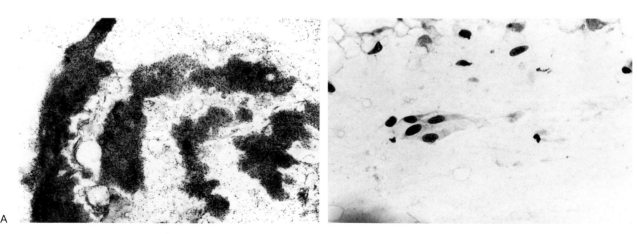

A

B

FIG. 3-15. Nodular fasciitis. **(A)** Numerous large fragments of tissue composed of spindle cells and inflammatory cells are present. The differential diagnosis would include fibromatosis and low-grade metaplastic spindle cell neoplasm. (Papanicolaou stain, ×20) **(B)** Single, bland spindle cells resembling fibroblasts are present in other areas of the aspirate. The biopsy diagnosis was nodular fasciitis. (Papanicolaou stain, ×100)

Fibrocystic Changes

Fibrocystic changes are a common finding, affecting more than half of women 30 to 50 years of age. These changes are a common cause of a mass lesion or mammographically detected lesion of the breast. Fibrocystic change encompasses a wide variety of histologic changes in the breast including fibrosis, cyst, apocrine metaplasia, sclerosing adenosis, and ductal hyperplasia.[62] Clinically, the patient may represent with localized or generalized lumpiness, which may vary with the menstrual cycle. The FNA specimens of fibrocystic changes may be hypocellular as a result of the fibrotic nature of the breast tissue. Other findings in the fine needle aspirates are varied, but the presence of foam cells, ductal epithelial cells, and apocrine cells suggests the diagnosis (Fig. 3-16).[63] Ductal epithelial cells in fibrocystic changes are usually arranged in tight honeycomb-like groups (Fig. 3-17). Bipolar or naked nuclei, which are believed to be of myoepithelial origin, are often present and are usually associated with benign disease.[64]

CYTOLOGIC FINDINGS IN FIBROCYSTIC CHANGES
- Variable cellularity
- Honeycomb epithelial sheets
- Bipolar (naked) nuclei
- Apocrine metaplasia
- Foam cells

Fibrocystic changes can be divided into two categories, nonproliferative and proliferative, based on the degree of ductal epithelial hyperplasia.[65-68] Fibrocystic changes with minimal proliferative change imply no increased risk for the development of subsequent invasive cancer. However, fibrocystic changes with evidence of moderate or greater ductal hyperplasia have an increased risk of cancer, depending on the severity of hyperplasia. Because the degree of epithelial hyperplasia found in breast biopsies is correlated with an increased risk of developing invasive cancer, it is possible that FNA may provide a relatively noninvasive method of identifying women at increased risk. It has been shown in a population of women with a history of breast cancer that random FNA exhibits significantly more proliferative changes than in a control population.[69,70] Cytologic features that identified atypical hyperplasia were increase nuclear area and perimeter, in addition to architectural features such as increased overlap of cells. These data suggest that FNA has promise for screening women but is not well accepted because the cytopathologic criteria for the diagnosis of proliferative breast disease are not well defined.[71,72] The criteria for the diagnosis of proliferative breast disease as described by Page, Dupont, and others relies to a significant degree on architectural features.[65,67,68] These features include swirling of the intraluminal epithelial cells, slit-like sublumens, and overlapping of the cells. Some investigators have proposed that

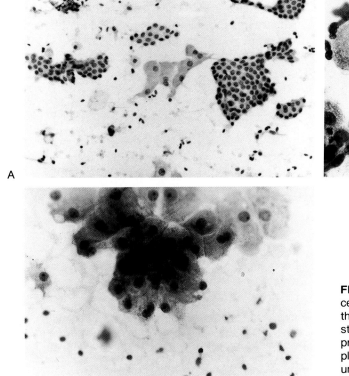
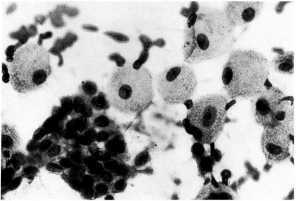

FIG. 3-16. Fibrocystic changes. (A) Benign epithelial cells, apocrine cells, and histiocytes are consistent with the diagnosis of fibrocystic changes. (Papanicolaou stain, ×100) (B) Numerous foamy histiocytes are often present. (Papanicolaou stain, ×200) (C) Apocrine metaplastic cells have abundant granular cytoplasm, round uniform nuclei, and single prominent nucleoli. (Papanicolaou stain, ×200)

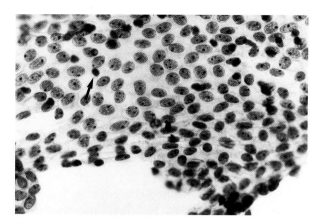

FIG. 3-17. Benign epithelial cells. This aspirate illustrates the flat, honeycomb appearance of benign epithelial cells. The scattered, oval, dark cells are myoepithelial cells (*arrow*), which are most often seen in benign lesions. (Papanicolaou stain, ×200)

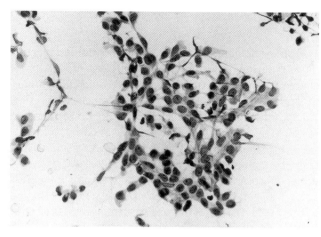

FIG. 3-19. Discohesive clusters. Although single epithelial cells are not usually prominent in fibrocystic changes, the clusters can show discohesion. (Papanicolaou stain, ×200)

these architectural features can be applied to evaluation of the fine needle aspirates, in addition to traditional cytopathologic criteria such as cellularity and nuclear morphology.[73,74] We studied 35 FNA smears of biopsy-confirmed hyperplasia to see if the architectural features described for the histologic diagnosis of proliferative breast disease could be applied to the aspirate smear.[73] In our study, the aspirates from proliferative breast disease had increased cellularity (Fig. 3-18), minimal atypia, and occasional discohesive epithelial clusters (Fig. 3-19). Many architectural features described for the histologic diagnosis of proliferative breast disease were observed in the aspirates. These architectural features can be best observed by focusing up and down through the epithelial clusters. The architectural changes include overlapping epithelial clusters with peripheral slit-like lumens (Fig. 3-20), and bulbous projections from the sublumen (Fig. 3-21). Myoepithelial cells were often observed in the ep-

ithelial clusters (Fig. 3-22). Because ductal carcinoma in situ (DCIS) is often in the differential diagnosis of an atypical hyperplasia and may thus represent the malignant end of the spectrum in proliferative breast disease, we compared the features observed in the proliferative disease cases with a series of DCIS in fine needle aspirates. In general, the DCIS cases had increased cellularity and atypia in comparison with the proliferative cases (Table 3-2). More importantly, distinct architectural differences were observed including the presence of rigid cribriform spaces with a lack of myoepithelial cells in DCIS. Sneige and colleagues also demonstrated that architectural features in fine needle aspirates are important in identifying proliferative changes and in differentiating from more worrisome lesions such as DCIS.[74,75]

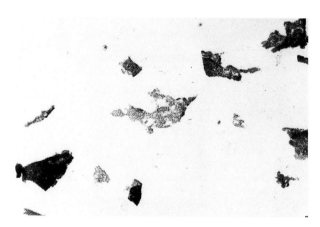

FIG. 3-18. Proliferative breast disease. Such changes often have increased cellularity in the FNA specimens. (Papanicolaou stain, ×20)

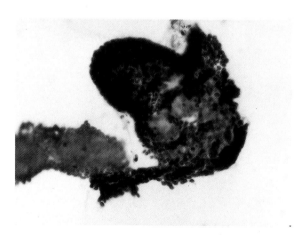

FIG. 3-20. Slitlike sublumens. This fine needle aspirate shows the irregular slitlike sublumens that may be present in proliferative breast disease. These sublumens are best observed by focusing up and down on overlapping, three-dimensional clusters of epithelial cells. (Papanicolaou stain, ×200)

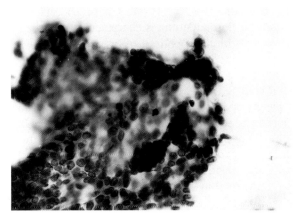

FIG. 3-21. Cellular projections. Small bulbous projections from the periphery of epithelial clusters are best appreciated by focusing through the cell group. (Papanicolaou stain, ×200)

CYTOLOGIC FINDINGS IN PROLIFERATIVE FIBROCYSTIC CHANGES

- Increased cellularity
- Sheets and clusters of cells with
    Slit-like sublumens
    Bulbous projections from the periphery
    Myoepithelial cells in groups

The differential diagnosis of fibrocystic changes cytologically often includes fibroadenoma and low-grade carcinoma (Fig. 3-23). Bottles and colleagues,[48] using stepwise regression analysis, found that stroma, staghorn clusters, and marked cellularity were the three most useful variables for distinguishing fibrocystic change in fibroadenomas. In fibrocystic changes, there were a greater number of honeycomb epithelial sheets and naked nuclei compared with ductal carcinomas.

Fibrocystic changes are part of a subset of benign lesions that can mimic carcinoma.[76] In these reported

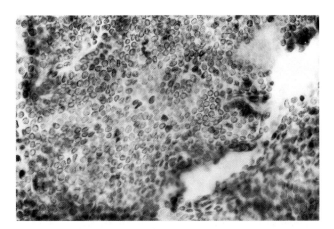

FIG. 3-22. Myoepithelial cells. In this slightly overlapping epithelial group, the oval to spindle-shaped dark cells are myoepithelial cells. The presence of these cells is often supportive of a benign lesion. (Papanicolaou stain, ×200)

TABLE 3-2. *Fibrocystic changes versus carcinoma in situ*

	Fibrocystic changes	Ductal carcinoma in situ
CYTOLOGIC CRITERIA		
Cellularity	Low to moderate	Moderate to high
Atypia	None to minimal	Moderate to marked
Nucleoli	Absent indistinct	Present
Single epithelial cells	None to few	Moderate
ARCHITECTURE		
Slitlike lumens	Prominent	Rare
Rigid lumens	Rare	Prominent
Intralumenal swirling	Present	Absent
Projections	Present	Rare
OTHER		
Myoepithelial cells	Prominent groups	Rare
Background	Clean	Necrosis/blood

cases, one clue that appears helpful to avoid a false-positive diagnosis is the presence of nuclei with a uniform chromatin pattern and small nucleoli.

BENIGN NEOPLASMS

Fibroadenoma

Fibroadenomas are the most common benign tumor of the breast. They occur most frequently in younger women but can occur at any age. They are usually solitary but may present as multiple lesions. Clinically, fibroadenomas present as round, mobile masses. Mammographically, they are often described as smoothly

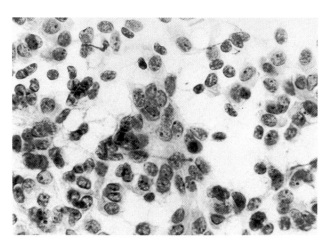

FIG. 3-23. Overlapping cytologic features of fibrocystic changes, fibroadenoma, and low-grade cancer. This aspirate is from a biopsy-confirmed fibroadenoma, an example of the overlapping features (single epithelial cells, increased cellularity, and atypia) that can be present in the FNA specimen. (Papanicolaou stain, ×200)

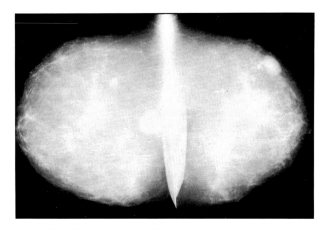

FIG. 3-24. Mammogram—fibroadenoma. This mammogram shows bilateral fibroadenomas that have smoothly outlined, round borders in both breasts.

outlined lesions (Fig. 3-24) (see Chap. 2).[77] The FNA specimen of fibroadenoma is characterized as a cellular aspirate with biphasic pattern of branching or staghorn epithelial clusters, bipolar (naked) nuclei, and stromal fragments (Fig. 3-25).[48,78,79] The branching pattern of epithelial cells is thought to be characteristic of, but not completely specific for, fibroadenoma. Bipolar (naked) nuclei can be seen within clusters and singly in the background. The epithelial cells from a fibroadenoma may be slightly enlarged but generally have a uniform fine chromatin pattern with indistinct or small nucleoli. The stromal fragments may have a striking myxoid appearance (Fig. 3-26).

CYTOLOGIC FINDINGS OF FIBROADENOMA

• Moderate to high cellularity
• Staghorn fragments of epithelial cells

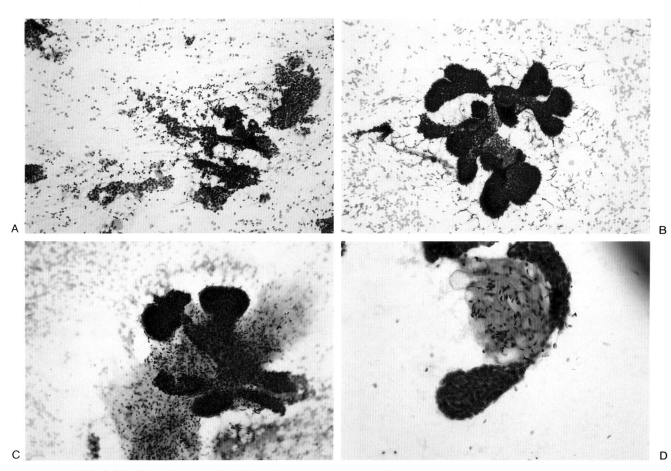

FIG. 3-25. Fibroadenoma. **(A)** A biphasic pattern consisting of staghorn epithelial clusters and numerous bipolar cells is most consistent with the diagnosis of fibroadenoma. (Papanicolaou stain, ×20) **(B)** The characteristic staghorn epithelial cluster that can be seen in fibroadenoma. (Papanicolaou stain, ×50) **(C)** Scattered fragments of stroma are helpful diagnostic clues in the FNA of fibroadenoma. (Papanicolaou stain, ×100) **(D)** In this aspirate, ductal epithelium is stretched around a stromal fragment. This is similar to the epithelial configuration seen in the histologic section. (Papanicolaou stain, ×100)

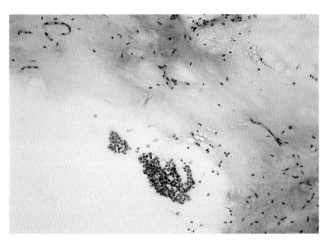

FIG. 3-26. Myxoid fibroadenoma. In this aspirate, abundant myxoid hypocellular stromal fragments were present. The biopsy confirmed the diagnosis of myxoid fibroadenoma. (Papanicolaou stain, ×100)

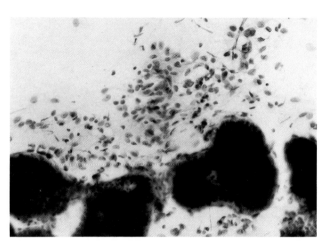

FIG. 3-28. Atypical fibroadenoma. The single epithelial cells in this fine needle aspirate from a fibroadenoma have a uniform, fine chromatin pattern and indistinct nucleoli. Benign epithelial fragments are present. (Papanicolaou stain, ×200)

- Stromal fragments
- Background of bipolar (naked) nuclei

With the appropriate clinical impression and the classic cytologic features on fine needle aspirates, the diagnosis of fibroadenoma can be readily made. However, fibroadenomas are often cited as a cause of false-positive diagnosis in cytology.[54] This is due to FNA specimens of fibroadenomas that have increased cellularity, including numerous single epithelial cells (Fig. 3-27) and nuclear atypia, which may be suggestive of a more serious lesion.[78] In these cases, it is important not to make a false cancer diagnosis. The finding of numerous myoepithelial cells and epithelial nuclei with a uniform fine chromatin pattern with small to indistinct nucleoli provides helpful clues to avoiding a false-positive diagnosis (Fig. 3-28). Bottles and colleagues reported that the most im-

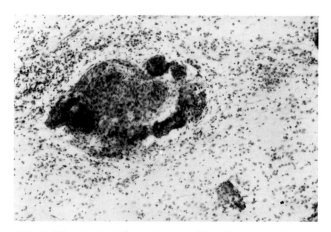

FIG. 3-27. Atypical fibroadenoma. The discovery of numerous single epithelial cells in an aspirate of a fibroadenoma can produce concern about a diagnosis of malignancy. The biopsy in this case confirmed the diagnosis of fibroadenoma. (Papanicolaou stain, ×100)

portant distinguishing cytologic features between fibroadenoma and ductal carcinoma were the presence of staghorn clusters, stroma, and honeycomb sheets.[48] Naked nuclei or myoepithelial cells even though they are classically as a prominent feature of benign lesions such as fibroadenoma, were not found to be a useful distinguishing feature in this study. The finding of bipolar (naked) cells in aspirates from malignant lesions has been described primarily in reports of the aspirate cytology of tubular carcinoma.[80] Many of the aspirates from tubular carcinoma resemble fibroadenomas or benign fibrocystic changes because of the presence of numerous bipolar (naked) nuclei in the background and benign epithelial cells. Even though a fine needle aspirate may have features consistent with a fibroadenoma when the features are atypical and include increased cellularity and epithelial discohesion, it is best to communicate this to the clinician and to recommend further diagnostic studies.

An important consideration in the differential diagnosis of the fine needle aspirate of fibroadenoma is the phyllodes tumor. Phyllodes tumors are a biphasic tumor composed of benign epithelial elements and a cellular stroma.[62,66] Histologically, the phyllodes tumor is distinguished from a fibroadenoma based on its leaflike pattern and cellular stroma. The distinction among benign, borderline, and malignant phyllodes tumors is based on the stromal cellular atypia and mitotic activity.[81-84] Cytologically, benign and borderline phyllodes tumors are similar to fibroadenoma and include numerous staghorn epithelial groups, bipolar cells, and stromal fragments. There may also be increased single stromal cells in the background. The degree of cellularity of the stromal fragments is increased in borderline and malignant tumors (Fig. 3-29). However, in benign phyllodes tumor, the stromal cellularity is similar to the fine needle aspirate findings in fibroadenomas.[81] Therefore, the distinction

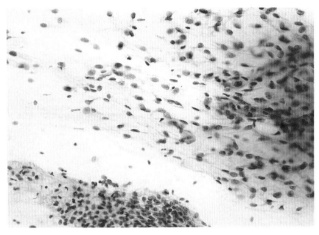

FIG. 3-29. Benign phyllodes tumor. Hypercellular stromal fragments. (Papanicolaou stain, ×50)

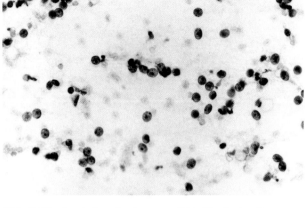

FIG. 3-31. Lactational adenoma. This illustrates the numerous, stripped nuclei with prominent nucleoli that may be present in a lactational adenoma. (Papanicolaou stain, ×200)

between a benign phyllodes tumor and a fibroadenoma can be difficult. Whenever hypercellular stromal fragments are present in fine needle aspirates that otherwise resemble a fibroadenoma, the diagnosis should suggest the possibility that these aspirates may be derived from a phyllodes tumor because these tumors may recur if not completely resected.

CYTOLOGIC FINDINGS IN PHYLLODES TUMOR
• Hypercellular stromal fragments
• Single plump stromal cells
• Epithelial clusters with features of hyperplasia
• Naked, bipolar cells

Lactational Adenoma

Most breast lesions in pregnant and postpartum patients are benign and are secondary to hormonal stimu-

lation by the pregnancy. FNA of these lesions produces a highly cellular aspirate composed of epithelial cells singly and in clusters with scalloped borders and granular, vacuolated cytoplasm (Fig. 3-30).[85–87] Stripped, single, round nuclei with large nucleoli may be prominent (Fig. 3-31). The background may have abundant granular material secondary to disruption of the delicate secretory cytoplasm (Fig. 3-32). The potential exists for a false cancer diagnosis in this setting owing to increased cellularity, cellular discohesion, and nuclei with prominent nucleoli. The criteria for malignancy for pregnant women are the same as for nonpregnant women.

CYTOLOGIC FINDINGS OF LACTATIONAL ADENOMA
• Cellular aspirate
• Ductal cells with granular, vacuolated cytoplasm
• Stripped nuclei with prominent nucleoli
• Granular, secretory background material

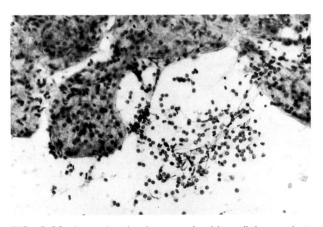

FIG. 3-30. Lactational adenoma. In this cellular aspirate, ductal epithelial cells with foamy, vacuolated cytoplasm and single "stripped" cells are present, consistent with the diagnosis of lactational adenoma. (Papanicolaou stain, ×100)

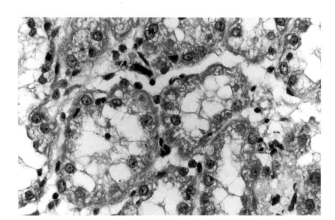

FIG. 3-32. Lactational adenoma. A histologic section from a lactational adenoma shows enlarged nuclei with prominent nucleoli and foamy, vacuolated cytoplasm. (Hematoxylin–eosin stain, ×200)

Uncommon Benign Neoplasms

Granular Cell Tumor

The granular cell tumor is an uncommon benign lesion that may mimic cancer clinically. These tumors present as firm to hard rounded nodules that may have infiltrative margins. These tumors are more commonly found in many other body sites, with granular cell tumors in the breast representing 6% to 8% of the total.[88] Fine needle aspirates of granular cell tumors are homogeneous and composed of loosely clustered cells with round nuclei and abundant eosinophilic granular cytoplasm. Prominent round nucleoli may be present. Cell borders often are indistinct (Fig. 3-33).[89]

CYTOLOGIC FINDINGS OF GRANULAR CELL TUMOR
- Cellular aspirate
- Cells in sheets and singly
- Uniform, round nuclei with abundant eosinophilic, granular cytoplasm

The differential diagnosis of granular cell tumor includes histiocytes derived from fat necrosis or trauma and apocrine carcinoma cells. The presence of a heterogeneous aspirate with an inflammatory component favors fat necrosis. Apocrine cancer exhibits pleomorphic nuclei and prominent irregular nucleoli, in addition to increased cellularity. Tumor cells are seen in clusters and singly, whereas granular cell tumors characteristically have increased single cells. Immunoperoxidase stains can also be helpful in the differential diagnosis. Granular cells are positive for S-100 protein and CD-68.[90]

Pleomorphic Adenoma

Pleomorphic adenoma is another uncommon benign lesion that can be seen using FNA of the breast.[91] The

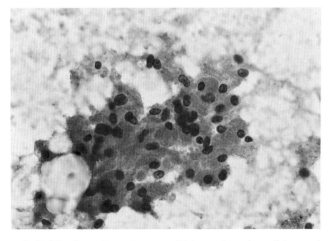

FIG. 3-33. Granular cell tumor. This aspirate is cellular and consists of numerous cells with abundant, eosinophilic granular cytoplasm. (Papanicolaou stain, ×200)

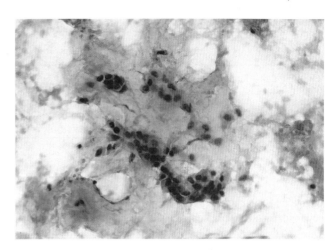

FIG. 3-34. Pleomorphic adenoma. Bland spindle- to oval-shaped myoepithelial cells are present. The background contains an abundant chondroid matrix that may be present in a mixed tumor. (Papanicolaou stain, ×100)

cytologic findings are similar, if not identical, to pleomorphic adenoma found in more common sites such as salivary gland. The aspirate may include myxoid to chondroid matrix material with clusters of bland myoepithelial type cells (Fig. 3-34). The differential diagnosis includes mucinous carcinoma and metaplastic carcinoma. In both of these malignancies, the epithelial cells should exhibit malignant cytologic features.

Adenomyoepithelioma

Adenomyoepithelioma is a rare benign tumor of myoepithelial cells that have the potential to recur.[92] These tumors are usually well circumscribed, round to multilobulated nodules. Histologically, their appearance ranges from spindle-shaped myoepithelial cells to a tubular pattern to a more solid lobulated pattern. There is limited experience with aspiration of these lesions; however, the cytologic findings that have been described include increased cellularity, numerous bipolar (naked) nuclei with occasional clusters of regular cohesive ductal cells with a rim of sentinel nuclei.[93]

MALIGNANT NEOPLASMS

Carcinoma In Situ

As the result of mammographic screening, DCIS is being detected at increasing frequency.[94] The diagnosis of DCIS implies a greater risk of the development of invasive cancer.[65,67] The histologic features of DCIS are variable but can be divided into two groups based on biologic behavior. Comedo DCIS, a subtype with more aggressive behavior, has high-grade nuclear features and central necrosis. Noncomedo carcinoma in situ has variable architectural features but has low-grade nuclei. The noncom-

TABLE 3-3. *Ductal carcinoma in situ*

Cytologic feature	Comedo DCIS	Noncomedo DCIS
Cellularity	Increased	Increased
Atypia	Marked	Minimal
Architecture	Sheets, clusters	Papillary fragments, cribriform
Diathesis	Extensive necrosis	Necrosis rarely seen

DCIS, ductal carcinoma in situ.

edo category includes the subtypes of micropapillary, cribriform, and solid carcinoma in situ.[95,96] It has been shown in several studies that FNA is limited in the diagnosis of carcinoma in situ because of its inability to distinguish between invasive and in situ cancers.[97—99] Most studies have looked at small numbers of cases and have grouped comedo and noncomedo DCIS subtypes together. If the two major groups are divided, it may be easier to distinguish a low-grade DCIS from invasive cancer. It has been suggested that there are distinguishing features between the two subtypes of comedo and noncomedo DCIS (Table 3-3).[100]

The cytologic findings in comedo-type carcinoma in situ are discohesive, pleomorphic enlarged tumor cells with irregular nuclei and often prominent macronucleoli.[101] The cells often have abundant cytoplasm and may be present in sheets or clusters or singly (Fig. 3-35). In comparison with cells of benign or atypical proliferative fibrocystic changes, the cytoplasm is more abundant and may be eosinophilic and granular.[102] The cell borders are often distinct. Extensive background necrosis is often present in the aspirates, and this may provide a useful clue to the diagnosis of comedo DCIS (Figs. 3-36 and 3-37). The aspirates of noncomedo DCIS have a cytologic pattern of increased cellularity with minimal

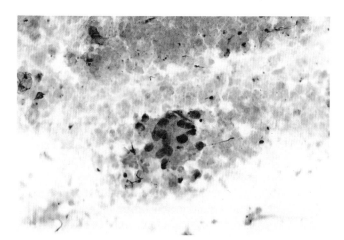

FIG. 3-36. Comedo ductal carcinoma in situ. This aspirate shows abundant background necrotic material, in addition to malignant cells. These features in the appropriate clinical setting suggest the diagnosis of comedo ductal carcinoma in situ. (Papanicolaou stain, ×100)

atypia.[98,101,102] The cells have uniform, slightly enlarged nuclei and small or indistinct nuclei. Architectural features include papillary fragments without distinct fibrovascular cores and epithelial groups with punched-out cribriform spaces or both (Fig. 3-38). This subtype generally lacks background necrosis. In both types of carcinoma in situ, myoepithelial cells are not a prominent feature in either the background or the epithelial clusters.[102]

Although carcinoma in situ can present as a palpable mass, it is more frequently nonpalpable with calcifications observed on mammographic screening. This clinical scenario, along with the cytologic findings, may allow the diagnosis of carcinoma in situ of either the comedo or noncomedo type to be suggested by FNA. In these

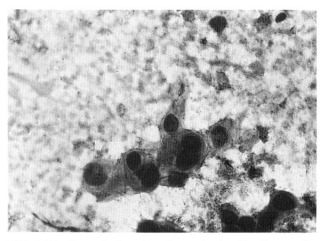

FIG. 3-35. Comedo ductal carcinoma in situ. The fine needle aspirate has clusters of cells with high-grade nuclear features. (Papanicolaou stain, ×200)

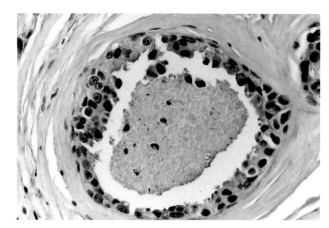

FIG. 3-37. Comedo ductal carcinoma in situ. The diagnostic features of comedo ductal carcinoma in situ of high-grade nuclei and central necrosis are illustrated. (Hematoxylin–eosin stain, ×100)

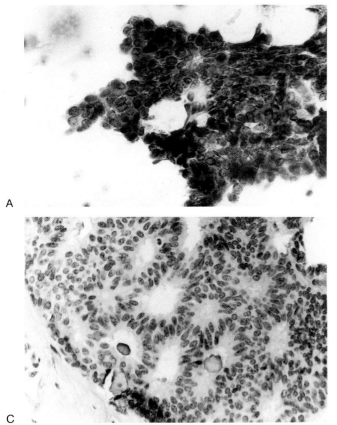

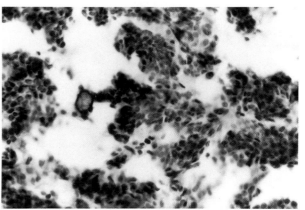

FIG. 3-38. Noncomedo ductal carcinoma in situ. (A) Minimal atypia and rigid cribriform spaces are illustrated in this photomicrograph. (Papanicolaou stain, ×200) (B) This shows increased cellularity with micropapillary fragments and microcalcifications. (Papanicolaou stain, ×100) (C) The biopsy corresponding to these two aspirates has prominent cribriform features with microcalcifications. (Hematoxylin–eosin stain, ×200)

cases, the possibility of invasive cancer must be ruled out on open surgical biopsy.

Lobular carcinoma in situ is characterized by small uniform cells filling and expanding lobular units. The presence of this lesion also implies an increased risk for the development of an infiltrating carcinoma. The diagnosis of lobular carcinoma in situ by FNA can be difficult because of the bland, small nature of the tumor cells.[54,103] The distinction between infiltrating lobular carcinoma and lobular carcinoma in situ has not been studied extensively, but it would be expected that differentiation is difficult.

Infiltrating Carcinoma

Infiltrating ductal carcinoma is the most commonly diagnosed breast cancer with an incidence of 75% to 85%. The diagnosis of infiltrating ductal carcinoma en-

compasses a wide variety of histologic and cytologic patterns. Histologically, the tumor cells may infiltrate in sheets, trabeculae, glands, and single cells. Often there is a desmoplastic stromal response to the tumor cells, which may result in a paucicellular fine needle aspirate.[66,104] Nuclear features range from bland (well differentiated) to pleomorphic (poorly differentiated). Many factors influence patient prognosis including the nuclear and histologic grade, presence of angiolymphatic invasion, and stage (size of tumor and lymph node status). By mammography, infiltrating ductal carcinoma is often seen as an ill-defined, stellate mass. The lesion feels hard by clinical examination and may have a gritty texture on aspiration.

The cytologic findings of infiltrating ductal carcinoma can be as varied as the histologic findings (Table 3-4).[63] Patterns that may be observed and diagnosed as malignancy in infiltrating ductal carcinoma include predomi-

TABLE 3-4. *General features of infiltrating carcinomas*

Cytologic feature	Infiltrating ductal	Infiltrating lobular
Cellularity	Moderate to high	Variable
Cell arrangement	Three-dimensional clusters, overlap	Molding, lining up
Single epithelial cells	Numerous	Moderate to numerous
Nuclear or cytoplasmic features	Nuclear enlargement, macronucleoli, chromatin clumping	Small hyperchromatic nuclei, small nucleoli, eccentric nuclei, vacuoles in cytoplasm

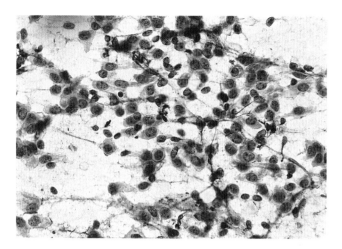

FIG. 3-39. Infiltrating ductal carcinoma—single-cell pattern. This aspirate consists predominantly of single cells with pleomorphic nuclei and small nucleoli. (Papanicolaou stain, ×200)

FIG. 3-41. Infiltrating ductal carcinoma—paucicellular. This aspirate is hypocellular, but the cells are discohesive and exhibit features of malignancy. (Papanicolaou stain, ×200)

nantly single epithelial cells (Fig. 3-39), clusters of malignant cells (Fig. 3-40), or paucicellular aspirates with highly malignant cells (Fig. 3-41). The cytologic nuclear features range from well differentiated with uniform small nuclei and fine chromatin (Fig. 3-42) to poorly differentiated with pleomorphic nuclei, clumped chromatin, and prominent nucleoli (Fig. 3-43). The recognized criteria for diagnosis of malignancy are (1) moderate to high cellularity; (2) three-dimensional epithelial or overlapping clusters; (3) the presence of numerous single epithelial cells; and (4) nuclear atypia including nuclear enlargement, macronucleoli, and chromatin clumping.[54,63] In general, it is important to observe all of the criteria of discohesion, increased cellularity, and nuclear atypia before a positive diagnosis of carcinoma is made because in some practices mastectomy is performed without frozen section confirmation. In our practice, we recommend frozen section confirmation before defini-

tive surgical therapy. Some of the protocols for preoperative chemotherapy accept positive FNA results for a diagnosis of breast cancer. If doubt exists, the FNA results should be called atypical or suggestive of carcinoma, and further diagnostic biopsy should be recommended, or the need for frozen section confirmation should be communicated to the clinicians involved.

Potential pitfalls for the diagnosis of infiltrating ductal carcinoma include cellular fibroadenomas with atypia (see Fig. 3-27), inflammatory lesions with marked reactive atypia (see Fig. 3-9), and lactational adenomas with increased cellularity (see Fig. 3-30). The cytologic features of these lesions have been discussed previously.

Infiltrating lobular carcinoma constitutes 5% to 10% of all invasive cancers. These tumors have an increased incidence of bilateralism and have a similar prognosis to infiltrating ductal cancers.[66] In the histologic section, small uniform cells infiltrate fibrous tissue singly and in

A

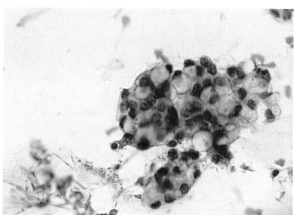

B

FIG. 3-40. Infiltrating ductal carcinoma—three-dimensional clusters and signet-ring cell differentiation. **(A)** Some cancers appear as overlapping, tight clusters with only minimal evidence of discohesion. (Papanicolaou stain, ×200) **(B)** This cluster of cells has prominent signet-ring cell differentiation. (Papanicolaou stain, ×200)

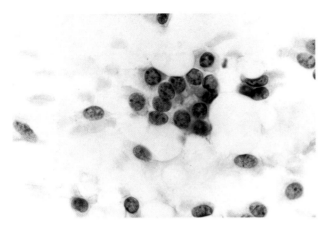

FIG. 3-42. Well-differentiated ductal carcinoma. These malignant cells are uniform with a fine chromatin pattern and indistinct nucleoli. (Papanicolaou stain, ×300)

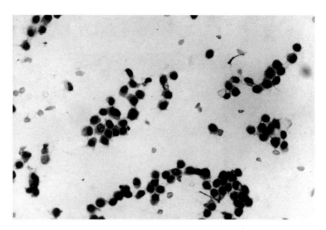

FIG. 3-44. Infiltrating lobular carcinoma. This aspirate is cellular, consisting primarily of single cells with small round nuclei. The nuclei are eccentrically placed in some cells. (Papanicolaou stain, ×50)

cords ("Indian file" pattern). The diagnosis of lobular carcinoma by FNA can be difficult. In many studies, this tumor accounts for a large number of false-negative diagnoses mainly because of its monotonous, bland cytologic features.[23,24] Other reasons for misdiagnosis include limited cellularity and minimal atypia such that the small tumor cells resemble lymphocytes. In addition, the tumor cells may be admixed in the adipose tissue and may be overlooked in the evaluation of the fine needle aspirate. The cytologic findings of lobular carcinoma consist of a low to moderately cellular aspirate with predominantly single cells (Fig. 3-44; see Table 3-4).[63,105] In most smears, the nuclei are small, uniform, and hyperchromatic with scant cytoplasm (Fig. 3-45). These tumor cells may be admixed in adipose tissue and difficult to detect. The nuclei may be eccentrically located with vacuoles in the cytoplasm (Fig. 3-46). Pleomorphic lobular cancer is a variant of lobular cancer with a high nuclear grade; it has a more aggressive course than classic lobular carcinoma. The tumor cells on aspirates show

nuclear enlargement, pleomorphism, and occasional prominent nucleoli.[106] The differential diagnosis includes ductal cancer, but the finding of small uniform cells and single filing of tumor cells may help to suggest the diagnosis.

The features of ductal and lobular carcinoma may overlap in the histologic section and in the fine needle aspirate. Some infiltrating carcinomas have characteristics of both ductal and lobular cancer. For this reason, many malignant aspirates are diagnosed as adenocarcinoma without specifying the type, unless classic features of a particular subtype of breast cancer are present. The distinction is not crucial for the FNA diagnosis, because the tumors are treated in a similar fashion.

Special Types of Cancer: Low-Grade Malignancies

The following tumors are distinct from one another but are similar in that they share a better prognosis than

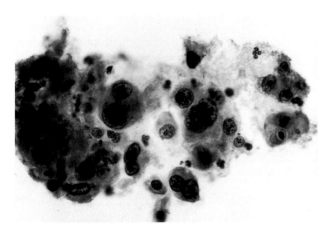

FIG. 3-43. Poorly differentiated ductal carcinoma. The tumor cells are markedly pleomorphic with clumped chromatin and prominent macronucleoli. (Papanicolaou stain, ×300)

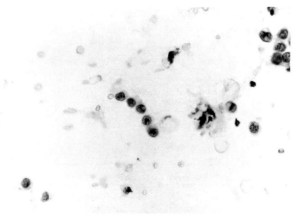

FIG. 3-45. Infiltrating lobular carcinoma. In this aspirate, the lobular carcinoma cells line up in single file, in a manner similar to that often observed in the histologic section. (Papanicolaou stain, ×100)

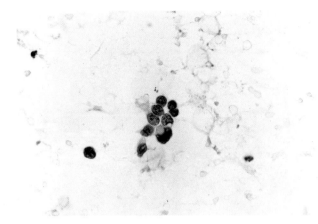

FIG. 3-46. Pleomorphic lobular carcinoma. The tumor cells in this fine needle aspirate exhibit pleomorphic features with nuclear irregularities and cytoplasmic vacuolization. Findings such as this may suggest the diagnosis of pleomorphic lobular carcinoma. (Papanicolaou stain, ×200)

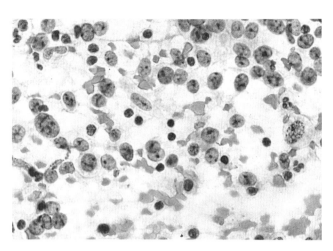

FIG. 3-47. Medullary carcinoma. A biphasic population of single malignant epithelial cells and lymphocytes is present. The features are suggestive of medullary carcinoma. (Papanicolaou stain, ×200)

infiltrating ductal and lobular cancer and they each constitute about 5% of all breast cancers. Although many of these tumors are not easily diagnosed by FNA because of their low-grade cytologic features, certain clues aid in their recognition (Table 3-5).

Medullary Carcinoma

Medullary carcinomas are unusual in that they have features of high-grade carcinoma (nuclear morphology) but have a less aggressive behavior.[107] They are usually well circumscribed and may be mistaken clinically and mammographically for a fibroadenoma. The FNA specimen of a medullary carcinoma is easily diagnosed as a malignancy. The specific cytologic findings that aid in the recognition of medullary carcinoma include a highly cellular aspirate with syncytial and numerous single tumor cells, large pleomorphic nuclei with macronucleoli, and a background of lymphocytes and plasma cells (Fig. 3-47).[108] In some cases, predominantly single epithelial cells are present and the differential diagnosis includes a lymphoma. The diagnosis of medullary carcinoma can be suggested based on the aspirate findings, but there may be overlap between the findings of infiltrating ductal carcinomas that have a prominent inflammatory infiltrate. The clinical picture in conjunction with the FNA

findings can help the cytopathologist to achieve the greatest specificity for the diagnosis of medullary carcinoma.

CYTOLOGIC FINDINGS IN MEDULLARY CARCINOMA

- Highly cellular aspirate
- Syncytial groupings, single cells
- Large, pleomorphic nuclei with macronucleoli
- Background of lymphocytes and plasma cells

Papillary Neoplasms

The incidence of papillary carcinoma is about 5%. Intracystic papillary carcinoma is a particular subtype that tends to occur in women over age 50 and has a favorable prognosis.[109,110] These papillary cancers are usually well-circumscribed, cystic masses with prominent hemorrhage. The distinction between benign and malignant papillary lesions is often difficult using FNA.[111-113] Both benign papillomas and malignant papillary cancers may have markedly increased cellularity with numerous single cells, two features that are typically associated with malignancy (Table 3-6). In addition, both benign and malignant papillary lesions may have minimal atypia, making the differentiation even more difficult. Some in-

TABLE 3-5. *Fine needle aspiration of low-grade carcinoma*

Cytologic feature	Mucinous cancer	Papillary cancer	Tubular cancer
Cellularity	Moderate to high	High	Low to moderate
Architecture	Clusters	Papillary	Angular groups
Atypia	Minimal	Minimal	Minimal
Single cells	Numerous	Numerous	Few
Background material	Mucin	Blood	Myoepithelial cells
Other	—	Hyperchromatic stratified cells	Can look like fibroadenoma

TABLE 3-6. *Fine needle aspiration of papillary neoplasms*

Characteristic	Papilloma	Papillary carcinoma
Cellularity	Moderate	High
Atypia	Minimal	Minimal
Single cells	Moderate	Numerous
Papillary fragments	Frequent	Frequent
Columnar cells	Numerous	Hyperchromatic, "piled up"
Apocrine metaplasia	Present	Absent

vestigators have observed more cellularity and single cells in malignant papillary lesions than in benign papillomas, but they have concluded that distinguishing benign from malignant lesions is difficult without overt malignant features. We studied the fine needle aspirates of 12 papillary carcinomas and 17 papillomas to determine whether cytologic findings existed that could suggest a correct diagnosis.[111] A common pattern among all of the papillary neoplasms was a cellular aspirate with complex fronds and single high columnar epithelial cells (Fig. 3-48). The two major differences between benign and malignant papillary lesions were increased cellularity and single epithelial cells observed in the papillary carcinomas. There was significant overlap in the degree of nuclear atypia and in the presence of papillary fragments between the papillomas and papillary carcinomas. A diagnostic clue that was present in several papillary carcinomas was the presence of columnar, hyperchromatic nuclei with stratification that were lining up on hypervascular cores (Fig. 3-49). This nuclear hyperchromasia and stratification was not seen in benign papillomas. Although not a significant distinguishing feature, the greatest nuclear atypia was observed in the invasive papillary carcinomas, followed by the intracystic papillary carcinomas, and then the papillomas (Fig. 3-50). Abundant hemosiderin-laden macrophages have been reported to be prominent in intracystic papillary cancers and such presence is most likely related to the cystic nature of the lesions (Fig. 3-51). The benign intraductal papillomas had a pattern of increased cellularity including single cells and papillary fragments with minimal atypia. The finding of apocrine metaplastic cells was only in benign intraductal papillomas, and this can allow the cytopathologist to suggest the diagnosis of papilloma (Fig. 3-52). One pitfall for the diagnosis of papillary carcinoma is the FNA of an infarcted intraductal papilloma. Such aspirates may have abundant necrosis and marked reactive atypia (Fig. 3-53). The presence of acute inflammation, however, should warrant a suspicious diagnosis instead of a malignant diagnosis. Subtle clues can allow cytopathologists to favor either benign or malignant diagnosis when faced with a papillary neoplasm. Because features overlap in most cases, it is best to wait for the open biopsy for the definitive diagnosis.

Mucinous (Colloid) Carcinoma

Mucinous or colloid carcinomas generally occur in older women. These tumors tend to be well circumscribed and soft. The lesions are composed of pools of extravasated mucin with clusters of carcinoma cells. Although tumor cells are usually bland, they may have high-grade cytologic features.[62] The cytologic features of mucinous carcinoma include low to moderate cellularity, three-dimensional clusters, and single epithelial cells with atypia and a background of mucinous material (Fig. 3-54).[114,115] The single tumor cells typically have small nuclei with indistinct nucleoli. Eosinophilic to vacuolated cytoplasm may be present and the nuclei may be eccentrically located (Fig. 3-55A). In some aspirates, the tumor cells originating from a mucinous carcinoma have high-grade nuclear features (see Fig. 3-55B). The background mucinous material is the hallmark of this lesion. The mucin stains metachromatically with Diff-Quik but can also be easily seen on the Papanicolaou-stained slides (Fig. 3-56A). Signet-ring cell differentiation may be seen (see Fig. 3-56B). Other lesions that may have a mucinous background include mucocele-like lesions, fibroadenomas, and papillomas of the breast.[116] However the constellation of increased cellularity, presence of single epithelial cells and an abundance of mucin can aid in the correct identification of a mucinous carcinoma.

CYTOLOGIC FINDINGS IN MUCINOUS CARCINOMA
- Variable cellularity
- Clusters of cells, single cells
- Uniform nuclei and small nucleoli
- Mucinous background

In the pure form, mucinous carcinoma has a very good prognosis. If mucinous carcinoma is admixed with infiltrating ductal carcinoma, the prognosis is that of the in-

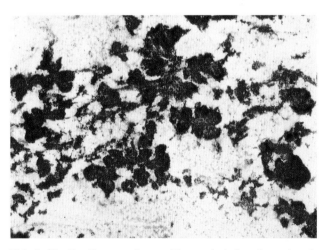

FIG. 3-48. Papillary carcinoma. The aspirate is extremely cellular and consists of cohesive, papillary fragments. (Papanicolaou stain, ×75)

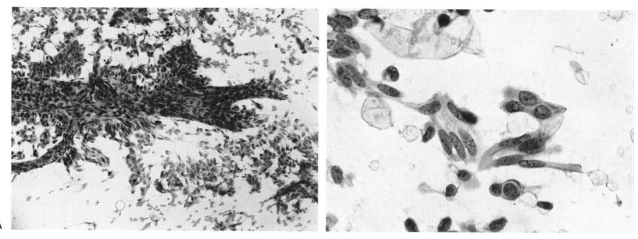

A   B

FIG. 3-49. Papillary carcinoma. **(A)** A large papillary fragment has stratified, with hyperchromatic cells lining up on a fibrovascular core. (Papanicolaou stain, ×100) **(B)** The columnar nature of the cells in a papillary carcinoma is illustrated in this aspirate. (Papanicolaou stain, ×200)

filtrating ductal cancer.[117] Morphometric studies have been performed to differentiate pure mucinous carcinomas (small cells) from mixed mucinous carcinomas (large cells), but no definite criteria have been described for FNA to distinguish between pure and mixed forms of mucinous carcinoma.

Tubular Carcinoma

Tubular carcinomas of the breast are usually small lesions detected by mammography and are often described as ill-defined and spiculated lesions.[118] The incidence of these tumors appears to be increasing secondary to detection by screening mammography. Mammographically, a small, ill-defined spiculated abnormality is the most common finding (Fig. 3-57). Patients with these

small, well-differentiated carcinomas have an excellent prognosis even in the presence of lymph node metastases. Histologically, bland nuclei forming angular glands infiltrate surrounding tissues in a haphazard manner (Fig. 3-58). The cytoplasm often has distinctive apocrine snouts. This low-grade carcinoma can be difficult to diagnose on FNA. Several reports have described FNA of tubular carcinoma in an attempt to find cytologic criteria to make this difficult diagnosis.[80,119,120] The following features have been reported to be helpful: increased cellularity with evidence of discohesion; nuclear atypia (generally minimal but may be moderate); and angular epithelial groups, which are characteristic, but not pathognomonic, of tubular carcinoma (Fig. 3-59). These features may be a minor component of the aspirate and require close scrutiny of the smear.[80] In many cases the

(text continues on page 43)

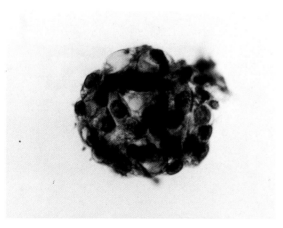

FIG. 3-50. Papillary carcinoma. Papillary cancers usually exhibit minimal atypia. This aspirate illustrates a cluster of cells from a papillary cancer that had moderate nuclear atypia. (Papanicolaou stain, ×200)

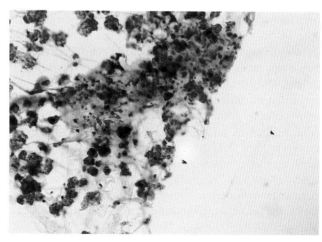

FIG. 3-51. Papillary carcinoma. Abundant hemosiderin-laden macrophages are seen in some aspirates of papillary carcinoma. (Papanicolaou stain, ×100)

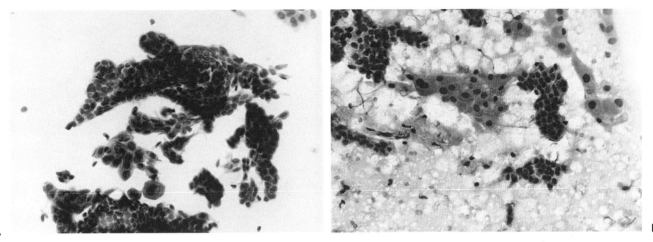

A   B

FIG. 3-52. Intraductal papilloma. This cellular aspirate had papillary fragments and evidence of apocrine metaplasia features associated with intraductal papilloma. (Papanicolaou stain, ×50)

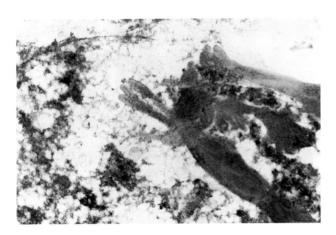

FIG. 3-53. Infarcted papilloma. Large necrotic papillary fragments and acute inflammation were present in this aspirate. Reactive epithelial atypia in this setting may lead to a diagnosis of malignancy. (Papanicolaou stain, ×100)

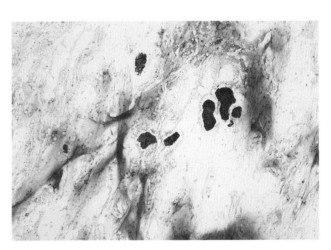

FIG. 3-54. Mucinous (colloid) carcinoma. Viewed on low power, this aspirate from a mucinous carcinoma has abundant mucin and rare clusters of malignant epithelial cells. (Papanicolaou stain, ×20)

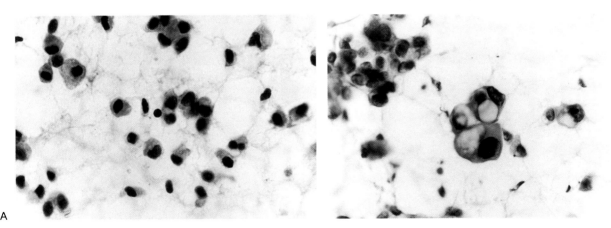

A   B

FIG. 3-55. Mucinous (colloid) carcinoma. **(A)** Typically, the nuclei in mucinous carcinoma are low grade with bland cytologic features. The nuclei are small and may be eccentrically placed in the cytoplasm. (Papanicolaou stain, ×200) **(B)** In some aspirates of mucinous carcinoma, high-grade nuclear features are present. This illustrates prominent signet-ring cell formation. (Papanicolaou stain, ×200)

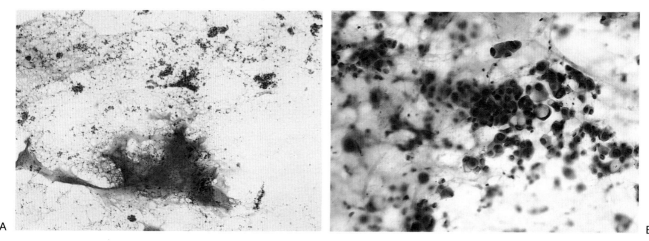

FIG. 3-56. Mucinous (colloid) carcinoma. (**A**) This aspirate shows the characteristic orange-magenta mucin noted on Papanicolaou stain. (×50) (**B**) Signet-ring cells can be observed in mucinous carcinoma. (Papanicolaou stain, ×200)

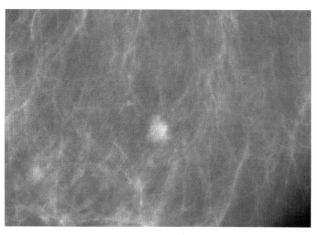

FIG. 3-57. Mammogram—tubular carcinoma. This mammogram illustrates a small, ill-defined spiculated lesion that is characteristic of a tubular carcinoma.

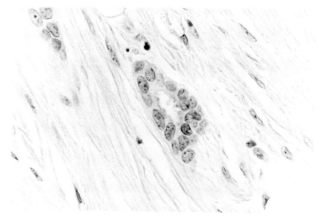

FIG. 3-58. Tubular carcinoma—histology. The characteristic angulated epithelial group with apocrine snouts and bland nuclear features is illustrated. (Hematoxylin–eosin stain, ×200)

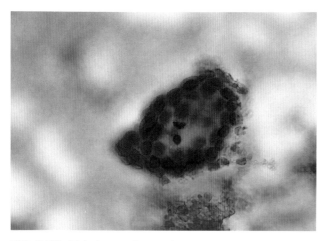

FIG. 3-59. Tubular carcinoma. In this aspirate, an angulated epithelial group is present that is identical to those seen in the histologic section. (Papanicolaou stain, ×300)

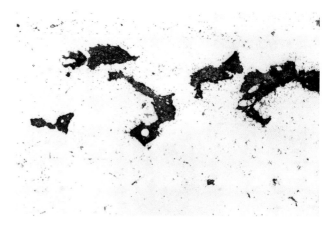

FIG. 3-60. Tubular carcinoma. On low power, the aspirate of a tubular carcinoma can look like a benign lesion with large, honeycomb epithelial sheets and bipolar cells in the background. (Papanicolaou stain, ×20)

aspirates resemble fibroadenomas or benign fibrocystic changes with staghorn epithelial groups and bipolar cells evident on low-power scan (Fig. 3-60), but on closer inspection in most cases discohesive angular epithelial groups with atypia and single epithelial cells were seen (Figs. 3-61 and 3-62). Myoepithelial cells, usually a hallmark of a benign lesion, have been described as a prominent component of the aspirate.[80,119,120] These benign-appearing findings may represent aspiration of adjacent hyperplastic ductal epithelium but such has not been proved. It is difficult to definitively make the diagnosis of tubular carcinoma on FNA, and most likely this difficulty is due to the small size of the lesions and the bland cytologic features. However, there are characteristic cytologic findings that allow the diagnosis to be suggested with subsequent confirmation by follow-up biopsy.

CYTOLOGIC FINDINGS IN TUBULAR CARCINOMA

- Low to moderately cellular aspirate
- Mild to moderate nuclear atypia
- Angular epithelial clusters
- Discohesive groups and scattered single cells

Cribriform carcinoma is another low-grade cancer that is in the differential diagnosis of tubular cancer. Quite frequently tubular and cribriform carcinomas have similar morphologic findings, and the histologic diagnosis is made based on the predominant component.[66] FNA findings in this tumor are not well described, but similar angular groups with the addition of epithelial groups with cribriform architecture would be present. The differential diagnosis from the mammographic findings would include the benign lesion, radial scar. Radial scars may have open angulated glands, thus making the differential diagnosis of tubular carcinoma difficult even in the histologic section. De la Torre and colleagues[119] compared the FNA findings of tubular cancers

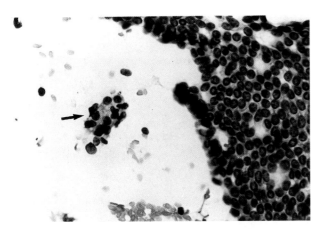

FIG. 3-61. Tubular carcinoma. A benign, honeycomb epithelial sheet is present. A cluster of atypical cells in an angular configuration provides a clue that this may be derived from a tubular cancer (*arrow*). (Papanicolaou stain, ×200)

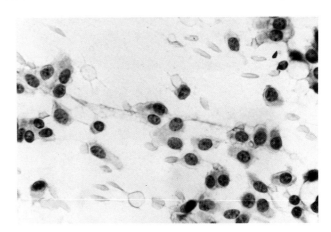

FIG. 3-62. Tubular carcinoma. Discohesive, single epithelial cells with bland cytologic features are present in this aspirate from a tubular carcinoma. (Papanicolaou stain, ×200)

and of radial scars. They found that although radial scar shared some of the features of tubular cancer, such as angular epithelial structures, it lacked features of atypia such as nucleoli and pleomorphism.

Unusual Malignant Lesions

Cystosarcoma Phyllodes

Cystosarcoma phyllodes is a biphasic stromal tumor with a benign epithelial component and a cellular spindle cell stroma.[62] The tumors are usually well-circumscribed fleshy masses with cystic areas. Generally, the stroma is more cellular than in a fibroadenoma. The distinction between a benign phyllodes tumor and a malignant cytosarcoma phyllodes is based upon increased stromal cellularity, mitotic activity, and anaplasia. In addition to benign and malignant categories of cystosarcoma phyllodes, a borderline (low malignant potential) category has been described. Mitotic activity is probably the most important distinguishing feature in differentiating benign from borderline phyllodes tumors.[121] The fine needle aspirate of cystosarcoma phyllodes tumors may have abundant sheets of epithelial cells with honeycomb, overlapping, and staghorn configurations.[122,123] Stromal fragments with increased cellularity should be present (Figs. 3-63 and 3-64). The cytologic features of malignant cystosarcoma phyllodes include isolated sarcomatous cells with pleomorphic nuclei and ill-defined cytoplasm, atypical highly cellular stromal fragments, and benign epithelial cells. Stromal cells are usually fibroblastic in origin; however, fat, cartilage, or bone differentiation may be found.[124] Phyllodes tumors can be diagnosed with FNA; however, the subtyping into benign, malignant, or borderline categories, unless definitive sarcomatous features are present, is best performed on the histologic section.[81,83,122]

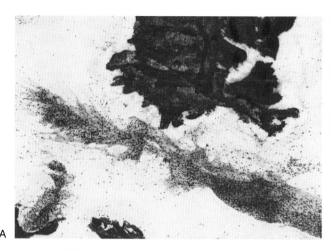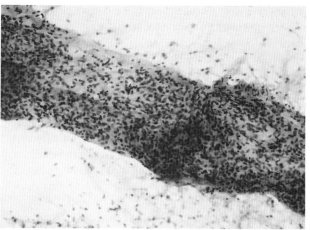

FIG. 3-63. Malignant cystosarcoma phyllodes. **(A)** Low-power view illustrating prominent staghorn epithelial groups and hypercellular stroma. (Papanicolaou stain, ×50) **(B)** The stroma exhibit marked hypercellularity with minimal atypia. The diagnosis of malignant cystosarcoma was based on increased mitotic activity in the biopsy. (Papanicolaou stain, ×100)

CYTOLOGIC FINDINGS IN MALIGNANT
CYTOSARCOMA PHYLLODES

- Cellular aspirate
- Abundant epithelial cells in sheets and overlapping
- Highly cellular stromal fragments
- Sarcomatous single cells

Metaplastic Carcinoma

Metaplastic carcinoma is a rare tumor, with an incidence of less than 1%, and has a poor prognosis. These neoplasms have a biphasic growth pattern with carcinomatous and sarcomatous elements.[124,125] Sarcomatous components such as spindle cell, squamous cell, bone, and cartilage with a high-grade epithelial component may be seen. Squamous differentiation may be found

(Fig. 3-65). Although usually high grade, low-grade spindle cell or metaplastic carcinomas have been described.[61,125] Cytologic features of metaplastic carcinoma include moderate to high cellularity, tumor diathesis or necrotic debris, and malignant cells, which may include epithelial and sarcomatous cells. Mesenchymal tissues such as bone and cartilage and benign multinucleated giant cells have been described in fine needle aspirate (Fig. 3-66).[123-129] In aspirates from a cartilage-producing tumor, the cartilaginous matrix can be easily identified on Diff-Quik–stained and Papanicolaou-stained slides (Figs. 3-67 and 3-68). In low-grade metaplastic carcinomas, the aspirate may have a population of atypical fibroblast-like cells with no distinct epithelial component (Fig. 3-69). In this instance, the differential diagnosis includes entities such as nodular fasciitis, a benign reactive condition, and fibromatosis of the breast.[59,60]

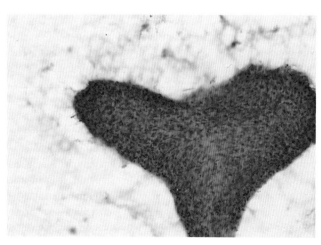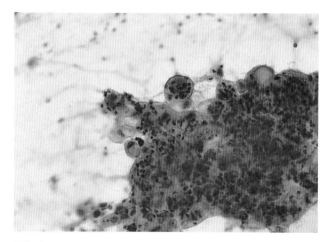

FIG. 3-64. Malignant cystosarcoma phyllodes. Another example of a hypercellular stromal fragment in an aspirate. The biopsy confirmed the diagnosis of malignant phyllodes tumor. (Papanicolaou stain, ×100)

FIG. 3-65. Metaplastic carcinoma with squamous features. This aspirate had clusters of pleomorphic cells with squamous features. (Papanicolaou stain, ×200)

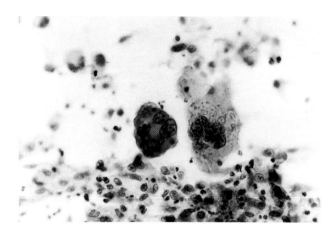

FIG. 3-66. Metaplastic carcinoma with giant cell features. Numerous giant cells with malignant features are present in this aspirate. (Papanicolaou stain, ×300)

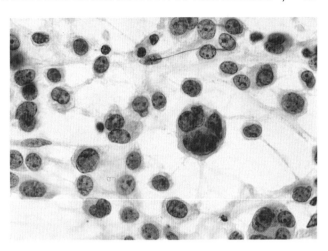

FIG. 3-68. Metaplastic carcinoma with cartilage. On high power, malignant chondrocytes and cartilaginous matrix are present. (Papanicolaou stain, ×200)

Pure sarcomas of the breast occur rarely. Malignant fibrous histiocytoma is one of the most common sarcomas of the breast. Other sarcomas include liposarcoma and angiosarcoma.[124] In general, the cytologic features are similar to those seen in aspirates of soft tissue tumors. Aspirates of liposarcoma may be paucicellular, but highly atypical lipoblasts may be found and are diagnostic.[130]

Apocrine Carcinoma

Apocrine carcinoma is an uncommon variant of infiltrating ductal carcinoma. These tumors resemble the cells of benign apocrine metaplasia, a common finding in fibrocystic changes (Fig. 3-70). Apocrine carcinoma is characterized by cells with abundant eosinophilic cytoplasm and large nuclei with prominent macronucleoli. This type of cancer does not have special prognostic sig-

nificance and is treated in a fashion similar to that of infiltrating ductal carcinoma.[66,131] The cytologic features include increased cellularity, single and clustered cells with apocrine features, and a necrotic diathesis in some cases (Fig. 3-71). The differential diagnosis includes a cellular aspirate of apocrine metaplasia. Features to make the distinction between apocrine carcinoma and abundant apocrine metaplasia are similar to those for diagnosing malignancy, that is, increased cellularity, nuclear atypia, and single epithelial cells.

CYTOLOGIC FINDINGS IN APOCRINE CARCINOMA

- Cellular aspirate
- Clusters and single cells
- Pleomorphic nuclei with prominent macronucleoli
- Abundant eosinophilic cytoplasm

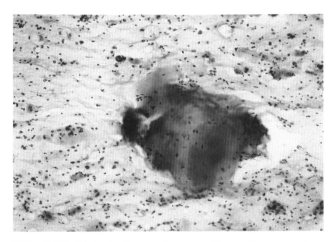

FIG. 3-67. Metaplastic carcinoma with cartilaginous features. This cellular aspirate had high-grade malignant cells and abundant cartilaginous matrix. (Papanicolaou stain, ×50)

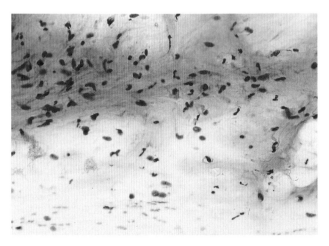

FIG. 3-69. Sarcoma. Atypical spindle cells with pleomorphic features and a myxoid background are present in this aspirate from a breast sarcoma with liposarcomatous features. (Papanicolaou stain, ×100)

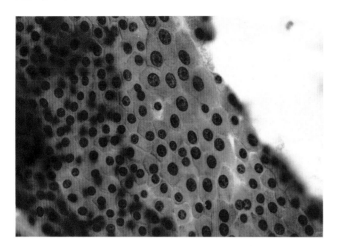

FIG. 3-70. Apocrine metaplasia. The features of apocrine metaplasia include abundant eosinophilic cytoplasm and round nuclei, which can have regular, prominent nucleoli. (Papanicolaou stain, ×200)

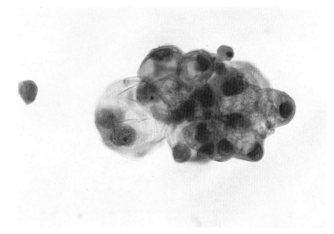

FIG. 3-72. Metastatic ovarian carcinoma. Clusters of large, malignant cells with vacuolated cytoplasm were present in this cyst fluid. The patient had a history of ovarian cancer, and the findings were consistent with origin from an ovarian cancer. (Papanicolaou stain, ×300)

Metastatic Carcinoma

Metastatic carcinoma of the breast is rare, with less than a 1% incidence.[132] These lesions may be well-circumscribed and freely movable. Primary tumors reported to be metastatic to the breast, in decreasing order of frequency, are melanoma, lymphoma, and ovarian and endometrial cancers.[133] Lung and prostate cancer metastatic to the breast have also been reported. The cytologic findings of metastatic breast cancer are similar to those of the primary site with the traditional criteria for malignancy. We have seen ovarian carcinoma metastatic to the breast with highly malignant cell clusters and vacuolated cytoplasm (Fig. 3-72). Renal cell carcinoma may have low-grade round nuclei with clear to granular cyto-

plasm (Fig. 3-73). The fine needle aspirate of metastatic melanoma may be highly cellular, with areas of pigment (Fig. 3-74). Hematopoietic neoplasms metastatic to breast yield aspirates composed of single monomorphic lymphoid cells the features of which are similar to the original lymphoma subtype (Fig. 3-75). Low-grade lymphomas can be difficult to diagnose by FNA and may require marker studies to confirm the diagnosis. For cases in which metastatic disease is suspected, the clinical history is of utmost importance. The diagnosis of a metastatic neoplasm often can be confirmed by comparing the cells on the aspirate with the original tumor. Immunoperoxidase stains can aid in the characterization of metastatic lesions; for example, melanoma markers (S-100, HMB-45) can confirm the diagnosis of melanoma.[62]

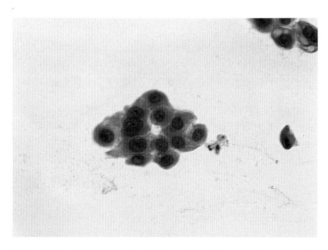

FIG. 3-71. Apocrine carcinoma. Apocrine carcinoma cells have abundant eosinophilic cytoplasm and pleomorphic nuclei with prominent nucleoli. (Papanicolaou stain, ×200)

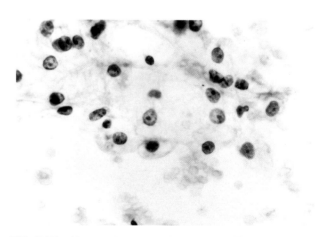

FIG. 3-73. Metastatic renal cell carcinoma. This aspirate had tumor cells with clear cytoplasm and round nuclei with nucleoli. The diagnosis of metastatic renal cell cancer was made in conjunction with the clinical history. (Papanicolaou stain, ×200)

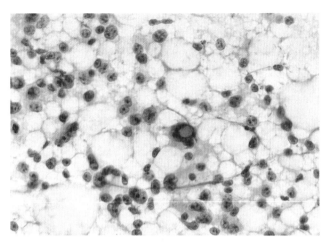

FIG. 3-74. Metastatic melanoma. The cells in this aspirate were discohesive with occasional bizarre cells. Melanin pigment was focally present. (Papanicolaou stain, ×200)

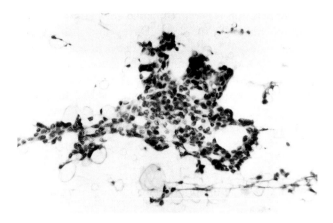

FIG. 3-76. Gynecomastia. This aspirate was moderately cellular and has benign epithelial fragments with overlap and features of ductal hyperplasia. (Papanicolaou stain, ×100)

FINE NEEDLE ASPIRATION OF THE MALE BREAST

Gynecomastia refers to enlargement of the male breast. It is fairly common; it is most often unilateral but may be bilateral. It has several causes, including drug use.[62,66] The cytologic findings of gynecomastia are moderate cellularity, tight multilayered epithelial groups, bipolar nuclei, and loosely adherent cells (Fig. 3-76).[134] On histologic section, gynecomastia often shows epithelial changes similar to those of severe to atypical ductal hyperplasia of the breast. These changes may be reflected in the aspirate by increased cellularity and mild to moderate architectural and nuclear changes.

Cancer of the male breast is usually of the infiltrating ductal type. It is uncommon, usually presenting as a painless mass.[134,135] Cytologic findings are similar to that seen with infiltrating ductal carcinoma in women.

SPECIAL STUDIES: APPLICATION TO BREAST FINE NEEDLE ASPIRATION

In the past, it has been acceptable to render a diagnosis of merely positive, suspicious, or negative for breast FNA. With increased reliance on FNA as a diagnostic procedure, it has become important to provide a specific diagnosis for both benign and malignant lesions, when possible.[136,137] A specific diagnosis of a particular subtype of cancer, such as a low-grade mucinous carcinoma, can guide therapy before a definitive surgical procedure. In addition to providing the maximum amount of diagnostic information from FNA, the usefulness of providing other prognostic information is an area of much interest. This prognostic information ranges from nuclear grading—an extension of the cytologic diagnosis—to special studies such as flow cytometry, immunocytochemical studies for tumor markers, and molecular diagnostic studies. Most of these techniques are currently being assessed as to their clinical usefulness; however, it is certain that in the future we will be able to provide even more information from the FNA specimen.

Nuclear Grade

One of the important prognostic features in breast cancer is the histologic and nuclear grade. Patients with well-differentiated tumors have a better survival rate than those with poorly differentiated tumors.[138] Although most of the studies of nuclear grade have been performed on histologic sections, fine needle aspirates are well suited for performing nuclear grading.[139-143] Alcohol-fixed, Papanicolaou-stained specimens have well-preserved nuclei with easily discerned chromatin patterns and nucleoli. Although few published studies of nuclear grade on FNA have correlated the cytologic nuclear grade with predictive prognostic value, it has

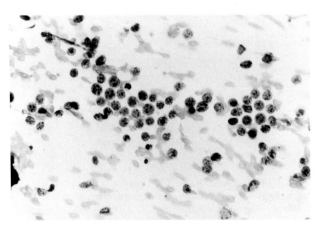

FIG. 3-75. Metastatic lymphoma. A homogenous population of small, noncleaved cells was present in this breast aspirate consistent with metastatic lymphoma. (Papanicolaou stain, ×200)

been shown that it is reproducible, correlating precisely with the histologic grade.[142] Davey and colleagues[141] have shown that it is feasible to perform nuclear grade and flow cytometry on fine needle aspirates with good correlation to the histologic nuclear grade. The method of nuclear grading that is generally used is the Fischer modification of the Black grading scheme.[144] With this method, three grades are used, with grade 1 representing well-differentiated tumors and grade 3 representing poorly differentiated tumors. Grade 1 nuclear features are characterized by small uniform nuclei with round, smooth nuclear membranes, fine chromatin, and indistinct nucleoli (Fig. 3-77A). These nuclei are generally derived from well-differentiated tumors such as tubular cancers. Nuclear grade 2 tumors have enlarged nuclei (and can be twice the size of grade 1), with smooth nuclear membranes, uniform chromatin, and small nucleoli (see Fig. 3-77B). Grade 3 nuclei have marked anisonucleosis, often with three-fold variation in nuclear diameter. There may be nuclear hyperchromatism with coarse chromatin and clearing. Macronucleoli are often identified (see Fig. 3-77C). The cytopathologist can aid in patient management at the level of the initial FNA in three ways: by diagnosing an aspirate as malignant; by subtyping the malignancy, if possible; and by assigning a nuclear grade to provide the maximum amount of information.[136,142,143] This information can be provided rapidly and cost effectively without performing any other special studies.

Steroid Receptors

The assessment of estrogen and progesterone receptors in breast cancer is standard practice as a guide to therapeutic options and prognostic information for the patient.[145,146] In recent years, the immunocytochemical detection of receptors has become accepted as a reproducible and accurate method of assessing receptor status.[147] This method offers the advantage of being able to see the tumor cells and assess the receptor status in the tumor cells instead of measuring receptor levels in normal breast cells. These immunocytochemical techniques can be applied to FNA of a breast malignancy to assess steroid receptor status.[145,148,149] Excellent correlation has been found between the immunocytochemistry on FNA specimens and immunocytochemical studies performed on the histologic biopsy specimens.[150] The sensitivity and specificity of the estrogen receptor immunocytochemistry on FNA samples range from 71% to 95% when

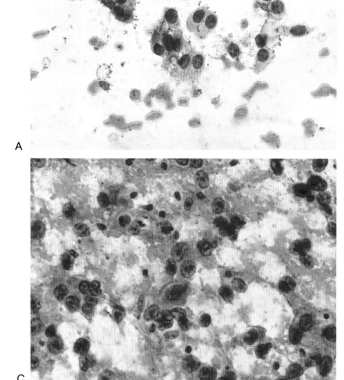

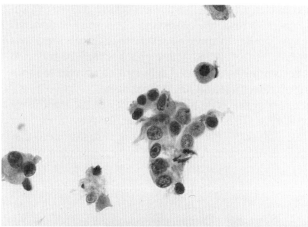

A

B

C

FIG. 3-77. Nuclear grade. **(A)** Nuclear grade I has uniform small nuclei with fine chromatin and inconspicuous nucleoli. (Papanicolaou stain, ×200) **(B)** Nuclear grade II has slight nuclear enlargement with chromatin changes and regular nucleoli. (Papanicolaou stain, ×200) **(C)** Nuclear grade III has pleomorphic enlarged nuclei with chromatin clumping, nuclear membrane irregularities, and macronucleoli. (Papanicolaou stain, ×200)

compared with the standard biochemical method.[151] The estrogen and progesterone receptor determination on FNA specimens is usually semiquantitated by counting the percentage of positive cells; however, image analysis methods that more objectively evaluate receptor stain intensity have been described.[152] Immunocytochemical studies for estrogen and progesterone receptors on FNA material are probably best suited for patients who have a small amount of tumor available, patients who can be treated preoperatively with chemotherapy based on the FNA diagnosis, and patients who refuse surgery.

Flow Cytometry and DNA Analysis

The clinical prognostic value of DNA analysis by flow and static cytometry is not well established. In select clinical situations, however, the information is used as a guide for therapeutic management. The DNA content of breast malignancies has been correlated with the histologic and nuclear grade, steroid receptor status, and stage.[153,154] Although most of these studies have been performed on fresh or paraffin-embedded tissue, both DNA flow and static cytometric techniques have been applied to FNA specimens with good correlation with tissue results.[155,156] The flow cytometric studies are performed on a suspension of cells stained with a fluorescent dye, which binds to the DNA. Static cytometric studies are performed on fixed cells on a slide and are usually stained with Feulgen, a dye that binds stoichiometrically to DNA (Fig. 3-78). Both DNA content and S-phase, an estimate of proliferation, can be determined from these studies on FNA specimens. The S-phase estimate has been found to be an important prognostic marker in certain subsets of patients. In combination with the DNA content information, the S-phase estimate can provide valuable clinical information. Flow cytometric studies are generally more accurate for S-phase estimate than

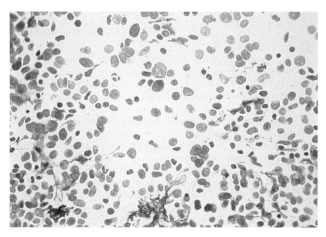

FIG. 3-78. Static cytometry—Feulgen method. Feulgen stains the DNA in the nucleus blue. (Feulgen method, ×100)

static cytometric studies because of the increased number of cells that can be analyzed in a short amount of time.[156,157] The development of more sophisticated image analysis equipment, however, may allow the more rapid analysis of numerous Feulgen-stained cells. If the breast FNA sample is to be used for DNA studies, it is helpful to have an initial rapid assessment to determine whether tumor is present, followed by additional FNA passes to obtain adequate cells.[33]

Proliferation and Other Tumor Markers

Proliferative activity of breast cancer has been shown to be correlated with prognosis using several different methods.[153,154,158,159] Several available antibodies recognize antigens associated with proliferative activity. Most of these have been studied on frozen or paraffin-embedded breast tissue, but proliferative markers have been applied to breast FNA specimens with success. Ki-67, a marker that is present on all cells that have entered the cell cycle, has been studied in FNA specimens.[158,159] These studies have found that the Ki-67 scores in FNA samples are lower than in frozen sections. Because the frozen section samples a small portion of the tumor and FNA samples a wider area in the tumor, it is possible that the Ki-67 staining in the FNA samples is more representative. One advantage to applying these proliferation markers to FNA specimens is that the nuclear stain can be more easily quantitated than in the tissue section, because cells are usually more dispersed over the slide.

Other tumor markers that have significance in the pathogenesis and prognosis of breast cancer have been applied to breast FNA specimens. Her-2/neu oncoprotein is a transmembrane protein with tyrosine kinase activity. Neu overexpression is associated with poor survival in patients with breast cancer.[160] Although numerous studies have looked at overexpression of neu by immunocytochemistry in frozen and paraffin-embedded tissue sections, only limited studies have looked at its expression in FNA specimens.[161] In one study, excellent correlation was found between detection of neu overexpression in FNA samples and in tissue sections, demonstrating the suitability of breast FNA for evaluation of neu overexpression. The tumor suppressor gene, p53, has been shown to be associated with poor prognosis in breast cancer.[162] Limited studies have described the immunocytochemical detection of p53 in FNA specimens and have shown that it is feasible on the FNA smears (Fig. 3-79).[163] These are just a few examples of markers that can be applied to the breast FNA specimen; many more will become available and will require carefully designed studies to determine their clinical usefulness.

These ancillary studies, ranging from simple nuclear grading performed on the Papanicolaou-stained smear

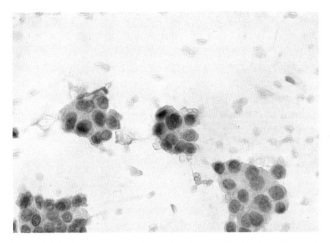

FIG. 3-79. Immunocytochemistry for p53. This breast aspirate has been stained immunocytochemically with antibody to p53. The nucleus is stained a dark red-brown. (Immunocytochemistry, ×200)

to more technically advanced studies such as flow cytometry, immunocytochemistry, and molecular diagnostics, are just beginning to find a role in FNA breast cytology. They offer, as will additional markers and molecular diagnostic studies, the opportunity to provide the most accurate diagnostic and prognostic information from the simple, rapid, relatively noninvasive procedure, FNA of the breast.

REFERENCES

1. Boring CC, Squires TS, Tong T. Cancer statistics, 1992. CA 1992; 42:19.
2. Feig SA. Decreased breast cancer mortality through mammographic screening: results of clinical trials. Radiology 1988;167: 659.
3. Harris J, Lippman ME, Veronesi U, et al. Breast cancer. N Engl J Med 1992;327:319.
4. Strax P. Detection of breast cancer. Cancer 1990;66:1336.
5. Winchester DP. Evaluation and management of breast abnormalities. Cancer 1990;66:1345.
6. McLelland R, Pisano ED. Issues in mammography. Cancer 1990; 66:1341.
7. Brenner RJ. Screening mammography. Cancer 1990;66:1348.
8. Martin HE, Ellis EB. Biopsy by needle puncture and aspiration. Ann Surg 1930;92:169.
9. Stewart FW. The diagnosis of tumors by aspiration biopsy. Am J Pathol 1933;9:801.
10. Frable WJ. Needle aspiration of the breast. Cancer 1984;53:671.
11. Frable WJ. Fine-needle aspiration biopsy. Hum Pathol 1983; 14:9.
12. Vetrani A, Fulciniti F, Di Benedetto G, et al. Fine-needle aspiration biopsies of breast masses: an additional experience with 1153 cases (1985 to 1988) and a meta-analysis. CA 1992;69:736.
13. Giard RWM, Hermans J. The value of aspiration cytologic examination of the breast. Cancer 1992;69:2104.
14. Zarbo RJ, Howanitz PJ, Bachner P. Interinstitutional comparison of performance in breast fine-needle aspiration cytology. Arch Pathol Lab Med 1991;115:743.
15. Deschenes L, Fabia J, Meisels A, et al. Fine needle aspiration biopsy in the management of palpable breast lesions. Can J Surg 1978;21:417.
16. Hammond S, Keyhani-Rofagha S, O'Toole RV. Statistical analysis of fine needle aspiration cytology: a review of 678 cases plus 4,236 cases from the literature. Acta Cytol 1987;31:276.
17. Layfield LJ, Parkinson B, Wong J, et al. Mammographically guided fine-needle aspiration biopsy of nonpalpable breast lesions: can it replace open biopsy? Cancer 1991;68:2007.
18. Bibbo M, Scheiber M, Cajulis R, et al. Stereotaxic fine needle aspiration cytology of clinically occult malignant and premalignant breast lesions. Acta Cytol 1988;32:193.
19. Logan-Young WW, Hoffman NY, Janus JA. Fine-needle aspiration cytology in the detection of breast cancer in nonsuspicious lesions. Radiology 1992;184:49.
20. Hann L, Ducatman BS, Wang HH, et al. Nonpalpable breast lesions: evaluation by means of fine-needle aspiration cytology. Radiology 1989;171:373.
21. Bell DA, Hajdu SI, Urban JA, et al. Role of aspiration cytology in the diagnosis and management of mammary lesions in office practice. Cancer 1983;51:1182.
22. Lannin DR, Silverman JF, Pories WJ, et al. Cost-effectiveness of fine needle biopsy of the breast. Ann Surg 1986;203:474.
23. O'Malley F, Casey TT, Winfield AC, et al. Clinical correlates of false-negative fine needle aspirations of the breast in a consecutive series of 1,005 patients. Surg Gynecol Obstet 1993;176:360.
24. Kreuzer G, Zajicek J. Cytologic diagnosis of mammary tumors from aspiration biopsy smears. III. Studies on 200 carcinomas with false-negative or doubtful cytologic reports. Acta Cytol 1972;16:249.
25. Hermansen C, Skovgarrd Poulsen H, Jensen J, et al. Diagnostic reliability of combined physical examination, mammography, and fine-needle puncture ("Triple-Test") in breast tumors. Cancer 1987;60:1866.
26. Kline TS, Joshi LP, Neal HS. Fine needle aspiration of the breast: diagnoses and pitfalls: a review of 3545 cases. CA 1979;44:1458.
27. Lamb J, Anderson TJ, Dixon MJ, et al. Role of fine needle aspiration cytology in breast cancer screening. J Clin Pathol 1987;40: 705.
28. Gent HJ, Sprenger E, Dowlatshahi K. Stereotaxic needle localization and cytological diagnosis of occult breast lesions. Ann Surg 1986;204:580.
29. Lofgren M, Anderson I, Lindholm K. Stereotactic fine-needle aspiration for cytologic diagnosis of nonpalpable breast lesions. AJR 1990;154:1191.
30. Fornage BD, Faroux MJ, Simatos A. Breast masses: US-guided fine-needle aspiration biopsy. Radiology 1987;162:409.
31. Rosenberg AL, Schwartz GF, Feig SA, et al. Clinically occult breast lesions: localization and significance. Radiology 1987;162: 167.
32. Cohen MB, Rodgers RPC, Hales MS, et al. Influence of training and experience in fine needle aspiration biopsy of breast: receive operating characteristics curve analysis. Arch Pathol Lab Med 1988;112:560.
33. Silverman JF, Lannin DR, O'Brien K, et al. The triage role of fine needle aspiration biopsy of palpable breast masses. Acta Cytol 1987;31:731.
34. Sickles EA. Periodic mammographic follow-up of probably benign lesions: results in 3,814 consecutive cases. Radiology 1991;179:463.
35. Bolmgren J, Jacobson B, Nordenstrom B. Stereotactic instrument for needle biopsy of the mamma. AJR 1977;129:721.
36. Dowlatshahi K, Yaremko ML, Kluskens LF, et al. Nonpalpable breast lesions: findings of stereotaxic needle-core biopsy and fine-needle aspiration cytology. Radiology 1991;181:745.
37. Schmidt RA: Stereotactic breast biopsy. CA 1994;44:172.
38. Jackson VP, Reynolds HE. Stereotaxic needle-core biopsy and fine-needle aspiration cytologic evaluation of nonpalpable breast lesions. Radiology 1991;181:633.
39. Elvecrog EL, Lechner MC, Nelson MT. Nonpalpable breast lesions: correlation of stereotaxic large-core needle biopsy and surgical biopsy results. Radiology 1993;188:453.
40. Gisvold JJ, Goellner JR, Grant CS, et al. Breast biopsy: a comparative study of Stereotaxically guided core and excisional techniques. AJR 1994;162:815.
41. Parker SH, Lovin JD, Jobe WE, et al. Stereotactic breast biopsy with a biopsy gun. Radiology 1990;176:741.

42. Parker SH, Jobe WE, Dennis MA, et al. US-guided automated large-core breast biopsy. Radiology 1993;187:507.

43. Casey TT, Rodgers WH, Baxter JW, et al. Stratified diagnostic approach to fine needle aspiration of the breast. Am J Surg 1992;163:305.

44. Mulford DK, Dawson AE. Atypia in fine needle aspiration cytology of nonpalpable and palpable mammographically detected breast lesions. Acta Cytol 1994;38:9.

45. Al-Kaisi N. The spectrum of the "gray zone" in breast cytology: a review of 186 cases of atypical and suspicious cytology. Acta Cytol 1994;38:898.

46. Stanley MW, Henry-Stanley MJ, Zera R. Atypia in breast fine-needle aspiration smears correlates poorly with the presence of a prognostically significant proliferative lesion of ductal epithelium. Hum Pathol 1993;24:630.

47. Peterse JL, Koolman-Schellekens MA, Van de Peppel-Van de Ham T, et al. Atypia in fine-needle aspiration cytology of the breast: a histologic follow-up study of 301 cases. Semin Diagn Pathol 1989;6:126.

48. Bottles K, Chan JS, Holly EA, et al. Cytologic criteria for fibroadenoma: a stepwise logistic regression analysis. Am J Clin Pathol 1988;89:707.

49. King EB, Chew KL, Hom JD, et al. Characterization by image cytometry of duct epithelial proliferative disease of the breast. Mod Pathol 1991;4:291.

50. Takeda T, Suzuki M, Sato Y, et al. Aspiration cytology of breast cysts. Acta Cytol 1980;26:37.

51. Ciatto S, Cariaggi P, Bulgaresi P. The value of routine cytologic examination of breast cyst fluids. Acta Cytol 1987;31:301.

52. Maygarden SJ, Novotny DB, Johnson DE, et al. Subclassification of benign breast disease by fine needle aspiration cytology. Acta Cytol 1994;38:115.

53. Goodson WH, Mailman R, Miller TR. Three year follow-up of benign fine-needle aspiration biopsies of the breast. Am J Surg 1987;154:58.

54. Kline TS. Masquerades of malignancy: a review of 4,241 aspirates from the breast. Acta Cytol 1981;25:263.

54a. Edmiston CE, Walker AP, Krepel CJ, et al. The nonpuereral breast infection: aerobic and anaerobic microbial recovery from acute and chronic disease. J Infect Dis 1990;162:695.

55. Adair FE, Munger JT. Fat necrosis of the female breast: report of 110 cases. Am J Surg 1947;74:117.

56. Habif D, Persin K, Lattes R. Subareolar abscess associated with squamous metaplasia. Am J Surg 1970;119:523.

57. Silverman JF, Lannin DR, Unverferth M, et al. Fine needle aspiration of subareolar abscess of the breast: spectrum of cytomorphologic findings and potential diagnostic pitfalls. Acta Cytol 1986;30:413.

58. Tabatowshi K, Elson CE, Johnston WW. Silicone lymphadenopathy in a patient with a mammary prosthesis: fine needle aspiration cytology, histology and analytical electron microscopy. Acta Cytol 1990;34:10.

59. Dahl I, Akerman M. Nodular fasciitis: a correlative cytologic and histologic study of 13 cases. Acta Cytol 1981;25:215.

60. Tani EM, Stanley MW, Skoog L. Fine needle aspiration cytology presentation of bilateral mammary fibromatosis. Acta Cytol 1988;32:555.

61. Gersell DJ, Katzenstein A-LA. Spindle cell carcinoma of the breast: a clinicopathologic and ultrastructural study. Hum Pathol 1981;12:550.

62. Tavassoli FA. Pathology of the breast. Norwalk, CT, Appleton & Lange, 1992:442.

63. Kline TS, Kline IK. Breast: guides to clinical aspiration biopsy. New York, Igaku-Shoin, 1989:35.

64. Tsuchiya S, Maruyama Y, Koike Y, et al. Cytologic characteristics and origin of naked nuclei in breast aspirate smears. Acta Cytol 1987;31:285.

65. Dupont WD, Page DL. Risk factors for breast cancer in women with proliferative breast disease. N Engl J Med 1985;312:146.

66. Page DL, Anderson TJ. Diagnostic histopathology of the breast. Edinburgh, Churchill Livingstone, 1987:341.

67. Dupont WD, Parl FF, Hartmann WH, et al. Breast cancer risk associated with proliferative breast disease and atypical hyperplasia. Cancer 1993;71:1258.

68. McDivitt RW, Stevens JA, Lee NC, et al. Histologic types of benign breast disease and the risk of breast cancer. Cancer 1992;69:1408.

69. Marshall CJ, Schumann GB, Ward JH, et al. Cytologic identification of clinically occult proliferative breast disease in women with a family history of breast cancer. Am J Clin Pathol 1991;95:157.

70. Skolnick MH, Cannon-Albright LA, Goldcar DE, et al. Inheritance of proliferative breast disease in breast cancer kindreds. Science 1990;250:1715.

71. Dziura BR, Bonfiglio TA. Needle cytology of the breast: a quantitative and qualitative study of the cells of benign and malignant ductal neoplasia. Acta Cytol 1979;23:332.

72. Marković-Glamočak M, Boban D, Sučić M, Oberman B, Sčukanec-Spoljar M. Significance of proliferative epithelial changes in breast fine-needle aspiration. Cancer 1992;70:781.

73. Dawson AE, Mulford DK, Sheils LA. The cytopathology of proliferative breast disease. Am J Clin Pathol 1994;103:438.

74. Sneige N, Staerkel GA. Fine needle aspiration cytology of ductal hyperplasia with and without atypia and ductal carcinoma insitu. Hum Pathol 1994;25:485.

75. Masood S, Frykberg ER, McLellan GL, et al. Cytologic differentiation between proliferative and non-proliferative breast disease in mammographically guided fine-needle aspirates. Diagn Cytopathol 1991;7:581.

76. Rogers LA, Lee KR. Breast carcinoma simulating fibroadenoma or fibrocystic change by fine-needle aspiration. Am J Clin Pathol 1992;98:155.

77. Tavasolli FA. Pathology of the breast. Norwalk, CT, Appleton & Lange, 1992:425.

78. Dejmek A, Lindholm K. Frequency of cytologic features in fine needle aspirates from histologically and cytologically diagnosed fibroadenomas. Acta Cytol 1991;35:695.

79. Maygarden SJ, Mc Call JB, Frable WJ. Fine needle aspiration of breast lesions in women aged 30 and under. Acta Cytol 1991;35:687.

80. Dawson AE, Logan-Young W, Mulford DK. Aspiration cytology of tubular carcinoma: diagnostic features with mammographic correlation. Am J Clin Pathol 1994;101:488.

81. Shimizu K, Masawa N, Yamada T, et al. Cytologic evaluation of phyllodes tumors as compared to fibroadenomas of the breast. Acta Cytol 1994;38:891.

82. Hart WR, Bauer RC, Oberman HA. Cytosarcoma phyllodes: A clinicopathologic study of 26 hypercellular periductal stromal tumors of the breast. Am J Clin Pathol 1978;70:211.

83. Simi U, Moretti D, Iacconi P, et al. Fine needle aspiration cytology pathology of phyllodes tumor: differential diagnosis with fibroadenoma. Acta Cytol 1988;32:63.

84. Silverman JF, Lannin DR, Frable WJ. Fine-needle aspiration cytology of mesenchymal tumors of the breast. Diagn Cytopathol 1988;4:50.

85. Novotny, DB, Maygarden SJ, Shermer RW, et al. Fine needle aspiration of benign and malignant breast masses associated with pregnancy. Acta Cytol 1991;35:676.

86. Bottles K, Taylor RN. Diagnosis of breast masses in pregnant and lactating women by aspiration cytology. Obstet Gynecol 1985;66:765.

87. Finley JL, Silverman JF, Lannin DR. Fine needle aspiration cytology of breast masses in pregnant women and lactating women. Diagn Cytopathol 1989;5:255.

88. Demay RM, Kay S. Granular cell tumor of the breast. Pathol Annu 1984;19:121.

89. Lowhagen T, Rubio C. The cytology of the granular cell myoblastoma of the breast. Acta Cytol 1977;21:314.

90. Ingram DL, Mossler JA, Snowhite J, et al. Granular cell tumors of the breast: steroid receptor analysis and localization of carcinoembryonic antigen, myoglobin and S-100 protein. Arch Pathol Lab Med 1984;108:897.

91. Diaz NM, McDivitt RW, Wick MR. Pleomorphic adenoma of the breast: a clinicopathologic and immunohistochemical study of 10 cases. Hum Pathol 1991;22:1206.

92. Tavassoli FA. Myoepithelial lesions of the breast: myoepitheliosis, adenomyoepithelioma and myoepithelial carcinoma. Am J Surg Pathol 1991;15:554.

93. Hock Ye-Lin, Chan Sui-Yum. Adenomyoepithelioma of the breast: a case report correlating cytologic and histologic features. Acta Cytol 1994;38:953.

94. Lagios MD, Westdahl PR, Morgolin FR, et al. Duct carcinoma in situ: relationship of extent of noninvasive disease to frequency of occult invasion, multicentricity, lymph node metastasis and short-term treatment failures. Cancer 1982;50:1309.

95. Schnitt SJ, Silen W, Sadowsky NL, et al. Ductal carcinoma in situ (intraductal carcinoma) of the breast. N Engl J Med 1988;318:898.

96. Ottesen GL, Graversent HP, Blichert-Toft M, et al. Ductal carcinoma in situ of the female breast. Am J Pathol 1992;16:1183.

97. Venegas R, Rutgers JL, Cameron BL, et al. Fine needle aspiration cytology of breast ductal carcinoma in situ. Acta Cytol 1994;38:136.

98. Wang HH, Ducatman BS, Eick D. Comparative features of ductal carcinoma in-situ and infiltrating ductal carcinoma of the breast on fine needle aspiration biopsy. Am J Clin Pathol 1989;92:736.

99. Abendroth CS, Wang HH, Ducatman BS. Comparative features of carcinoma in situ and atypical ductal hyperplasia of the breast on fine-needle aspiration biopsy specimens. Am J Clin Pathol 1991;96:654.

100. Malamud YR, Ducatman BS, Wang HH. Comparative features of comedo and non-comedo ductal carcinoma in-situ of the breast on fine needle aspiration biopsy. Diagn Cytopathol 1992;8:571.

101. Sneige N. Current issues in fine-needle aspiration of the breast: diagnostic problems of in-situ, lobular and ductal carcinomas and clinical implications of nuclear grading. In: Schmidt W, ed. Cytopathology annual. Baltimore, Williams & Wilkins, 1992:155.

102. Dawson AE, Mulford DK, Sheils LA. Cytologic feature of ductal carcinoma in-situ: a histologic and mammographic correlative study. Acta Cytol 1994;38A:802.

103. Salhany KE, Page DL. Fine needle aspiration of mammary lobular carcinoma in situ and atypical lobular hyperplasia. Am J Clin Pathol 1989;92:22.

104. Rosen PP. The pathological classification of human mammary carcinomas: past, present and future. Annu Clin Lab Sci 1979;9:144.

105. Antoniades K, Spector HB. Similarities and variations among lobular carcinoma cells. Diagn Cytopathol 1987;3:55.

106. Dabbs DJ, Grenko RT, Silverman JF. Fine needle aspiration of pleomorphic lobular carcinoma of the breast: duct carcinoma as a diagnostic pitfall. Acta Cytol 1994;34:923.

107. Maier WP, Roseman GP, Goldman LJ, et al. A ten-year study of medullary carcinoma of the breast. Surg Obstet Gynecol 1977;144:695.

108. Wargotz ES, Silverberg SG. Medullary carcinoma of the breast: a clinicopathologic study with appraisal of current diagnostic criteria. Hum Pathol 1988;19:1340.

109. Kraus FT, Neubecker RD. The differential diagnosis of papillary tumors of the breast. Cancer 1962;15:444.

110. Squires JE, Betsill WL. Intracystic carcinoma of the breast: a correlation of cytomorphology, gross pathology, microscopic pathology and clinical Data. Acta Cytol 1981;25:267.

111. Dawson AE, Mulford DK. Benign versus malignant papillary neoplasms of the breast: diagnostic clues in fine needle aspiration cytology. Acta Cytol 1994;38:23.

112. Jeffrey PB, Ljung BM. Benign and malignant papillary lesions of the breast: a cytomorphologic study. Am J Clin Pathol 1994;101:500.

113. Dei Tos AP, Della Giustina D, Bittesini L. Aspiration biopsy cytology of malignant papillary breast neoplasms. Diagn Cytopathol 1992;8:580.

114. Duane GB, Kanter MH, Branigan T, Chang C. A morphologic and morphometric study of cells from colloid carcinoma of the breast obtained by fine needle aspiration: distinction from other breast lesions. Acta Cytol 1987;31:742.

115. Gupta RK, Mc Hutchison AGR, Simpson JS, et al. Value of fine needle aspiration cytology of the breast, with an emphasis on the cytodiagnosis of colloid carcinoma. Acta Cytol 1991;35:703.

116. Ro JY, Sneige N, Sahin AA, et al. Mucocelelike tumor of the breast associated with atypical ductal hyperplasia or mucinous carcinoma. Arch Pathol Lab Med 1991;115:137.

117. Norris HJ, Taylor HB. Prognosis of mucinous (gelatinous) carcinoma of the breast. Cancer 1965;18:879.

118. Oberman HA, Fidler WJ. Tubular carcinoma of the breast. Am J Surg Pathol 1979;13:387.

119. de la Torre M, Lindholm K, Lindgren A. Fine needle aspiration cytology of tubular breast carcinoma and radial scar. Acta Cytol 1994;38:884.

120. Bondeson L, Lindholm K. Aspiration cytology of tubular breast carcinoma. Acta Cytol 1990;34:15.

121. Noris HJ, Taylor HB. Relationship of histologic features to behavior of cystosarcoma phyllodes. Cancer 1967;20:2090.

122. Dusenbery D, Frable WJ. Fine needle aspiration cytology of phyllodes tumor: potential diagnostic pitfalls. Acta Cytol 1992;36:215.

123. Rao CR, Narasimhamurthy NK, Jaganathan K, et al. Cystosarcoma phyllodes: diagnosis by fine needle aspiration cytology. Acta Cytol 1992;36:203.

124. Pollard SG, Marks PV, Temple LN, et al. Breast sarcoma: a clinicopathologic review of 25 cases. Cancer 1990;66:941.

125. Jebsen PW, Hagmar BM, Nesland JM. Metaplastic breast carcinoma: a diagnostic problem in fine needle aspiration biopsy. Acta Cytol 1991;35:396.

126. Boccato P, Briani G, d' Atri C, et al. Spindle cell and cartilaginous metaplasia in a breast carcinoma with osteoclastlike stromal cells: a difficult fine needle aspiration diagnosis. Acta Cytol 1988;32:75.

127. Gupta RK, Naran S, Fauck R, et al. Carcinoma of the breast with malignant epithelial giant cells: needle aspiration cytology, immunocytochemistry and electron microscopy in a rare case in a woman under 30. Acta Cytol 1992;36:430.

128. Gupta RK, Holloway LJ, Wakefield SJ, et al. Fine needle aspiration cytology, immunocytochemistry and electron microscopy in a rare case of carcinoma of the breast with malignant epithelial giant cells. Acta Cytol 1991;35:412.

129. Gorczyca W, Olszewski W, Tuziak T, et al. Fine needle aspiration cytology of rare malignant tumors of the breast. Acta Cytol 1992;36:918.

130. Foust RL, Berry AD, Moinuddin SM. Fine needle aspiration cytology of liposarcoma of the breast. Acta Cytol 1994;38:957.

131. Abati AD, Kimmel M, Rosen PP. Apocrine mammary carcinoma: a clinicopathologic study of 72 cases. Am J Clin Pathol 1990;94:371.

132. Hadju SI, Urban JA. Cancers metastatic to the breast. Cancer 1972;29:1691.

133. Silverman JF, Feldman PS, et al. Fine needle aspiration cytology of neoplasms metastatic to the breast. Acta Cytol 1987;31:291.

134. Gupta RK, Naran S, Simpson J. The role of fine needle aspiration cytology (FNAC) in the diagnosis of breast masses in males. Eur J Surg Oncol 1988;14:317.

135. Hecht JR, Winchester DJ. Male breast cancer. Pathology Patterns 1994;102(4):S25.

136. Sneige N, Staerkel GA, Caraway NP, et al. A plea for uniform terminology and reporting of breast fine needle aspirates: the MD Anderson Cancer Center proposal. Acta Cytol 1994;38:971.

137. Katz RL. A turning point in breast cancer cytology reporting: moving from callowness to maturity. (Editorial) Acta Cytol 1994;38:881.

138. Elston CW, Ellis IO. Pathological prognostic factors in breast cancer. I. The value of histologic grade in breast cancer: experience from a large study with long term follow-up. Histopathology 1991;19:403.

139. Ducatman BS, Emery ST, Wang HH. Correlation of histologic grade of breast carcinoma with cytologic features on fine-needle aspiration of the breast. Mod Pathol 1993;6:539.

140. Zajdela A, De LaRiva LS, Ghossein NA. The relation of prognosis to the nuclear diameter of breast cancer cells obtained by cytologic aspiration. Acta Cytol 1979;23:75.

141. Davey DD, Banks ER, Jennings D, et al. Comparison of nuclear grade and DNA cytometry in breast carcinoma aspirates to histologic grade in excised cancers. Am J Clin Pathol 1993;99:708.

142. Dabbs D. Role of nuclear grading of breast carcinomas in fine needle aspiration specimens. Acta Cytol 1993;37:361.

143. Hunt CM, Ellis ID, Elston CW, et al. Cytologic grading of breast cancer: a feasible proposition? Cytopathology 1990;1:282.

144. Fisher ER, Redmond C, Fisher B. Histologic grading of breast cancer. Pathol Annu 1980;15:239.
145. Masood S. Estrogen and progesterone receptors in cytology: a comprehensive review. Diagn Cytopathol 1992;8:475.
146. Osborne CK, Yochmowitz MG, Knight WA III, et al. The value of estrogen and progesterone receptors in the treatment of breast cancer. Cancer 1984;46:2884.
147. King WJ, DeSombre ER, Jensen EV, et al. Comparison of immunocytochemical and steroid-binding assays for estrogen receptor in human breast tumors. Cancer Res 1985;45:293.
148. Lundy J, Lozowski M, Sadri D, et al. The use of fine needle aspirates of breast cancer to evaluate hormone receptor status. Arch Surg 1990;125:174.
149. Nizzoli R, Bozzetti C, Savoldi L, et al. Immunocytochemical assay of estrogen and progesterone receptors in fine needle aspirates from breast cancer patients. Acta Cytol 1994;38:933.
150. Katz RL, Patel S, Sneige N, et al. Comparison of immunocytochemical and biochemical assays for estrogen receptor in fine needle aspirates and histologic sections from breast: carcinoma patients. Breast Cancer Res Treat 1990;15:191.
151. Silverman JF. Breast. In: Bibbo M, ed. Comprehensive cytopathology. Philadelphia, WB Saunders, 1991:761.
152. Franklin WA, Bibbo M, Doria MI, et al. Quantitation of estrogen receptor content and ki-67 staining in breast carcinoma by the microTICAS image analysis system. Anal Quant Cytol Histol 1987;9:279.
153. Auer G, Eriksson E, Azavedo E, et al. Prognostic significance of nuclear DNA content in mammary adenocarcinomas in humans. Cancer Res 1984;44:394.
154. Dressler LG, Seamer LC, Owens MA, et al. DNA flow cytometry and prognostic factors in 1331 frozen breast cancer specimens. Cancer 1988;61:420.
155. Klemi PJ, Joensuu H. Comparison of DNA ploidy in routine fine needle aspiration biopsy samples and paraffin-embedded tissue samples. Anal Quant Cytol Histol 1988;10:195.
156. Palmer JO, McDivitt RW, Stone KR, et al. Flow cytometric analysis of breast needle aspirates. Cancer 1988;62:2387.
157. Fuhr JE, Kattine AA, Nelson HS. Evaluation of in vivo breast fine needle aspirates by flow cytometry: an efficacy study. J Natl Cancer Inst 1992;84:1272.
158. Barnar NJ, Hall PA, Lemoine NR, et al. Proliferative activity in breast carcinoma determined in situ by Ki-67 immunostaining and its Relationship to clinical and pathologic variables. J Pathol 1987;152:287.
159. Kuenen-Boumeester V, Van Der Kwast Th H, Van Laarhoven HAJ, et al. Ki-67 staining in histological subtypes of breast carcinoma and fine-needle aspiration smears. J Clin Pathol 1991;44: 208.
160. Slamon DJ, Clark GM, Wong SG, et al. Human breast cancer: correlation of relapse and survival with amplification of the Her-2/neu oncogene. Science 1987;235:177.
161. Martin AW, Davey DD. Comparison of immunoreactivity of neu oncoprotein in fine needle aspirates and paraffin-embedded materials. Diagn Cytopathol 1995;12:142.
162. Ostrowski JL, Sawan A, Henry L, et al. p53 expression in human breast cancer related to survival and prognostic factors: an immunohistochemical study. J Pathol 1991;164:75.
163. Koutselini H, Malliri A, Field JK, et al. p53 expression in cytologic specimens from benign and malignant breast lesions. Anticancer Res 1991;11:1415.

Fine Needle Aspiration of Subcutaneous Organs and Masses,
edited by Yener S. Erozan and Thomas A. Bonfiglio.
Lippincott-Raven Publishers, Philadelphia, © 1996.

CHAPTER 4

Fine Needle Aspiration of the Lymph Nodes

Nancy P. Caraway and Ruth L. Katz

One of the earliest reports of the cytologic diagnosis of lymph node enlargement by means of fine needle aspiration (FNA) dates back to the beginning of the 20th century when Grieg and Gray[1] used it to diagnose trypanosomes in lymph nodes of Ugandan patients with sleeping sickness. Subsequently, in the early 1920s Guthrie[2] reported its use in cases of infectious etiology such as tuberculosis and syphilis lymphadenitis, as well as Hodgkin's disease, myeloid leukemia, and metastatic tumors. Today, indications for FNA of lymph nodes include (1) differentiating between a lymphoid process and an epithelial abnormality or metastasis involving a lymph node; (2) distinguishing patients with benign lymphadenopathy who can be followed clinically from those who have a lymphoproliferative abnormality that requires lymph node excision; (3) staging lymphoma; (4) selecting a lymph node for surgical excision; (5) documenting relapse; (6) documenting transformation to a higher grade lymphoma; (7) diagnosing deep sites to obviate the need for laparotomy, particularly in surgically high-risk patients; and (8) obtaining additional material for ancillary studies in patients who already have an established histologic diagnosis.[3]

The use of FNA to document metastatic tumors to lymph nodes has become a well-established diagnostic procedure associated with a high degree of accuracy.[4-6] In a recent study of lymphadenopathy in 1103 patients, Steel and colleagues[7] showed that the overall accuracy of FNA in identifying benign and malignant conditions was 96%; however, the accuracy for lymphomas, which numbered 139 in total, dropped to 72% compared with 96% for epithelial neoplasms. The major pitfall in this series, as well as other reported series, has been the difficulty in differentiating low-grade lymphoid neoplasia from reactive hyperplasia on FNA smears based solely on cytomorphology.

COLLECTION AND PREPARATION TECHNIQUES

The technique of acquiring adequate material to perform ancillary studies has been previously described but will be briefly summarized.[8-10] The lymph node is sampled using a fine (25-gauge) needle with or without aspiration. Immediate assessment of the specimen allows the pathologist to determine whether an atypical lymphoid population is present. Adequate material can usually be procured for ancillary studies in three to four passes. A small drop of the concentrated specimen is smeared on glass slides, and the remainder of the specimen is rinsed in a preservative solution that can be later subdivided for

N. P. Caraway and R. L. Katz: Department of Pathology,
Section of Cytology, The University of Texas, MD Anderson
Cancer Center, Houston, Texas 77030.

ancillary studies. Although we routinely perform immunophenotyping on cytospin preparations, and in some instances by flow cytometry, we realize that not all laboratories are able to perform these studies. In these instances, the material can be procured and sent to a commercial or reference laboratory.

Cytospin preparations for marker studies are made from the lymphoid cells that are collected in a preservative media and concentrated by a simple density gradient centrifugation technique. A panel of at least four immunomarkers (kappa, lambda, CD3, and Ki-67) is initially made, and additional cytospins can be made in the event that further studies are needed. Immunomarkers can also be determined by flow cytometry. DNA ploidy analysis can be performed by flow cytometry or image analysis. A minimum of 10 million cells is needed for most of these studies, and this amount can usually be obtained in three to four passes. Molecular studies require 5 to 10 million cells and are performed only if a T-cell process is suspected or the immunophenotyping is inconclusive for lymphoma.

COMPLICATIONS OF LYMPH NODE FINE NEEDLE ASPIRATION

Complications from FNA biopsy are usually minor except for a rare event of significant hematoma or pneumothorax following aspiration of a supraclavicular or high-axillary lymph node. Histologic changes associated with the needle tract have been reported in a small percentage of surgically excised lymph nodes.[11-13] Depending on the time elapsed since the FNA procedure, these changes ranged from recent hemorrhage and necrosis to loose aggregates of lymphocytes, neutrophils, hemosiderin-laden histiocytes, fibrin, proliferating capillaries, spindle cells, and fibrosis. In less than 1% of cases, segmental infarction or coagulative necrosis was reported. Postaspiration infarction should be differentiated from spontaneous infarction, which occurs rarely in untreated patients with underlying lymphoma.[14] Theoretically, the incidence of complications can be reduced by using a thin needle (25 gauge), performing rapid iterative movements in one direction instead of multiple directions, and holding pressure after the procedure.[15]

REACTIVE LYMPH NODES AND LYMPHADENITIS

Aspirates of reactive lymph nodes are characterized by a polymorphous lymphoid population that in the proper clinical context may allow a confident diagnosis and obviate the need for an excisional biopsy. If an infectious process is suspected, aspirated material can be rinsed in sterile saline and cultured for microorganisms. Smears for special stains (Gram, Ziehl-Neelsen, Fite, Gomori

methenamine-silver stains) may be obtained at the time of FNA biopsy. If the lymph node does not show signs of regression following observation or antibiotic therapy within a few weeks, then an excisional biopsy is recommended.

Reactive Lymphoid Hyperplasia

The cytologic features of reactive hyperplasia vary, depending on the size of the germinal centers, the degree of stimulation, and whether the sample is derived primarily from the germinal center, interfollicular area, or paracortical tissues. Aspirates typically show a mixed population of lymphoid cells including small and large cleaved cells, large noncleaved cells, immunoblasts, and plasma cells that represent the full spectrum of transformation (Fig. 4-1). There is usually a subpopulation of small lymphoid cells that, depending on the evolution of the reactive process, may vary from a low to high percentage of the total cell population. Admixed with the lymphoid cells are variable numbers of tingible body macrophages, histiocytes, endothelial cells, eosinophils, and neutrophils. Although the presence of tingible body macrophages favors a reactive process, it does not exclude lymphoma (Fig. 4-2).

Although there is a mixture of small to large lymphoid cells in florid hyperplasia, atypical intermediate and large cells usually predominant. The increased number of mononucleated or binucleated atypical cells may be worrisome for lymphoma.

Immunophenotyping typically shows a polyclonal population (Fig. 4-3) with the absence of light-chain restriction kappa/lambda ratio of 3:1 or less. Reactive T cells may constitute a large component, but if they ex-

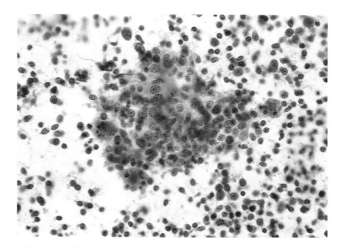

FIG. 4-1. Reactive lymphoid hyperplasia. Lymph node aspirate shows an aggregate of small and large follicular center cells and tingible body macrophages. (Papanicolaou stain, ×400)

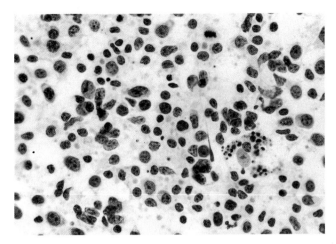

FIG. 4-2. Reactive lymphoid hyperplasia. A polymorphous population is seen composed of small and large cleaved cells, immunoblasts, plasmacytoid lymphocytes, and tingible body macrophages. (Papanicolaou stain, ×500)

ceed 80%, a low-grade T-cell lymphoma should be considered.

Cytokinetic studies usually show a diploid cell population with variable proliferative activity. Minor aneuploid populations and extremely high proliferative activities have occasionally been reported in patients infected with human immunodeficiency virus (HIV).[16]

The differential diagnosis of follicular hyperplasia includes mixed small cleaved and large cell lymphoma, large cell lymphoma, and T-cell lymphoma. Distinguishing mixed small cleaved and large cell lymphoma and follicular hyperplasia may be difficult on smears; however, the former lacks a well-defined transition of small to large cells and contains two discrete (one small and one large) subpopulations. In lymphoma, plasma cells

and tingible body macrophages are usually few in number or are absent. Large cell lymphoma may be considered when there is a florid proliferation of immunoblasts. Immunophenotyping is usually helpful in separating follicular hyperplasia from lymphoma. T-cell lymphomas containing plasma cells, eosinophils, and histiocytes may be mistaken for a reactive process. In some cases, molecular studies may be necessary to demonstrate T-cell derivation, particularly in low-grade T-cell lymphomas.

Suppurative Lymphadenitis

Initially in suppurative lymphadenitis there is an admixture of neutrophils and lymphoid cells. This is followed by purulent material composed of neutrophils and cellular debris (Fig. 4-4). Later, as the acute inflammatory process subsides, neutrophils are admixed with lymphocytes, plasma cells, and tingible body macrophages.

Granulomatous Lymphadenitis

The characteristic feature of granulomatous lymphadenitis is epithelioid histiocytes in a lymphoid background. Epithelioid cells have elongated, comma-shaped nuclei with finely granular chromatin and pale cytoplasm with indistinct cell borders (Fig. 4-5). The epithelioid cells may be loosely aggregated or form cohesive clusters reminiscent of granulomas in histologic sections. Multinucleated foreign-body or Langhans giant cells with nuclei peripherally arranged are variably present. Granulomatous lymphadenitis may or may not have associated necrosis, which appears as acellular granular material on smears.

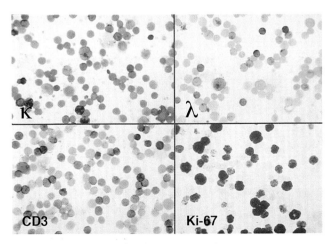

FIG. 4-3. Reactive lymphoid hyperplasia. Immunocytochemical studies show the following positive percentages: kappa 30%, lambda 30%, and CD3 40%, consistent with a reactive lymph node. Ki-67 shows a labeling index of 80%, which is high, but which can be seen in a reactive process. (Immunoperoxidase stain, ×500)

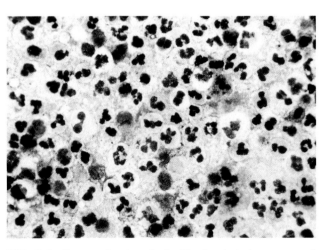

FIG. 4-4. Suppurative lymphadenitis. Aspirate is composed primarily of acute inflammatory cells and cellular debris. (Papanicolaou stain, ×500)

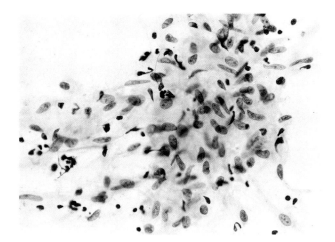

FIG. 4-5. Granulomatous lymphadenitis. Smear shows a cluster of epithelioid histiocytes and scattered lymphocytes from a patient with tuberculosis. (Papanicolaou stain, ×400)

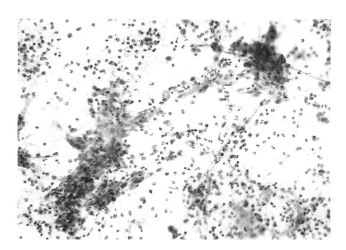

FIG. 4-6. Cat scratch disease. Axillary lymph node aspirate shows acute inflammatory cells, lymphocytes, and epithelioid histiocytes. (Papanicolaou stain, ×200)

Specific Types of Lymphadenitis

Bacterial Lymphadenitis

Bacteria, commonly staphylococci, may infect regional superficial lymph nodes that drain a dental abscess, appendicitis, tuboovarian abscess, or infected wound, causing a suppurative lymphadenitis.[17] Cat scratch disease caused by a gram-negative bacilli should be suspected if the aspirate contains numerous neutrophils admixed with epithelioid histiocytes and cellular debris (Fig. 4-6), particularly in an axillary node of a young patient who has had close contact with a cat. Lymphogranuloma venereum should be considered when suppurative granulomas involve inguinal lymph nodes.

Mycobacterial Lymphadenitis

Mycobacterium tuberculosis, atypical mycobacteria including *Mycobacterium avium-intracellulare*, and *Mycobacterium leprae* may affect lymph nodes. Smears of tuberculosis lymphadenitis may contain epithelioid histiocytes with or without necrosis or show only necrotic material and neutrophils without epithelioid histiocytes.[18,19] The presence of acid-fast bacilli in aspiration smears varies. Negative images of bacilli on air-dried Romanowsky stained smears may be helpful in detecting mycobacterial organisms.[20,21] One should think of *Mycobacterium avium-intracellulare* when there are aggregates of large histiocytes with negatively stained linear cytoplasmic inclusions resulting from the numerous intracytoplasmic bacilli (Fig. 4-7), particularly in immunosuppressed patients.[16] In addition to the histiocytes, neutrophils and necrosis are often present. In lepromatous leprosy, the characteristic cell is a syncytial histiocyte (Virchow cell or globus cell) with vacuolated cytoplasm containing numerous lepra bacilli. Gupta and col-

leagues[22] studied lymph node aspirates in cases of leprosy and described four cytologic types. They observed a progressive increase in the number of lymphocytes from types I to IV, with a change from the classic foamy histiocytes in types I and II to epithelioid histiocytes in type IV.

Fungal Lymphadenitis

Histoplasma capsulatum, *Coccidioides immitis*, and *Cryptococcus neoformans* may affect lymph nodes. Histoplasmosis and coccidioidomycosis are endemic in the central and southwestern regions of the United States, respectively. Lymph node aspirates of histoplasmosis show epithelioid histiocytes, lymphocytes, and necrosis; small (2 to 5 μm) narrow-based budding yeast forms are present within histiocytes and giant cells. Lymph node aspirates of coccidioidomycosis also show a necrotizing

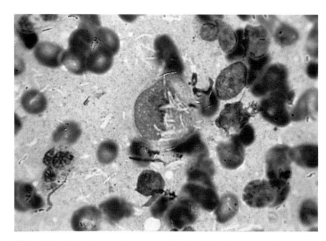

FIG. 4-7. Mycobacterium lymphadenitis. Negative image bacilli are present in histiocytes and in the background. (Diff-Quik stain, ×1000)

granulomatous process. A careful search may reveal thick-walled cysts and endospores. *C neoformans* is one of the few fungi that may affect both immunocompetent and immunosuppressed patients.[23] When it involves the lung and regional lymph nodes, it is referred to as a primary pulmonary lymph node complex of cryptococcosis.[24] Aspirates show epithelioid histocytes, yeast-filled giant cells, and lymphocytes (Figs. 4-8 and 4-9). The narrow-based budding yeasts have a thick mucopolysaccharide capsule that stains strongly positive with mucicarmine (Fig. 4-10).[25] Gomori methenamine-silver stain is helpful in detecting fungi on cytologic preparations. Coexisting infections with *C neoformans* and *Pneumocystis carinii* have been reported.[26]

Viral Lymphadenitis

Viruses that commonly affect the lymph nodes include the Epstein-Barr virus (infectious mononucleosis), cytomegalovirus, HIV, measles, varicella, and herpes. Aspirates of a viral lymphadenitis vary greatly. Usually there is a polymorphous population of atypical lymphocytes, plasmacytoid cells, plasma cells, immunoblasts, and multinucleated cells. The atypical lymphocytes have enlarged nuclei with fine nuclear chromatin, variably prominent nucleoli, and either a narrow rim of basophilic or relatively abundant cytoplasm. In infectious mononucleosis, the immunoblastic proliferation may be so florid that it may be misinterpreted as malignant lymphoma. Stanley and colleagues[27] emphasize that the single most important feature that distinguishes infectious mononucleosis from lymphoma is the spectrum of immunoblastic maturation in cells with plasmacytoid features. Binucleated immunoblast cells resembling Reed-Sternberg cells of Hodgkin's disease have occasionally been seen in infectious mononucleosis and postvaccinal

lymphadenitis;[27,28] however, most of these cells do not meet the strict criteria of Reed-Sternberg cells.

HIV lymphadenitis may show a spectrum of changes ranging from florid lymphoid hyperplasia to marked lymphoid depletion.[29,30] As in other viral lymphadenitis, aspirates typically show a heterogeneous population of small, intermediate, and large lymphocytes; plasma cells; and tingible body macrophages.[16,26,31,32] Oertel and colleagues[31] observed that the number of immunoblasts was higher in HIV lymphadenitis than in aspirates of hyperplasia from patients not infected with HIV. In some cases of florid hyperplasia, the presence of an increased number of large atypical cells may be worrisome for mixed small cleaved and large cell lymphoma or large cell lymphoma (Fig. 4-11). Most cases can be distinguished by immunophenotyping, but in rare instances of HIV lymphadenitis, the large atypical cells do not demonstrate positivity for kappa, lambda, or CD3, thereby making a definitive diagnosis difficult.[16,26]

Protozoal Lymphadenitis

Toxoplasma spp are believed to be the etiologic agents in 5% to 15% of cases of unexplained lymph node enlargement. The posterior cervical lymph nodes are most commonly affected, but other cervical, supraclavicular, and occipital lymph nodes may be involved.[17] Aspirates show a polymorphous lymphoid population, loosely aggregated epithelioid histiocytes, and tingible body macrophages. The crescent-shaped organisms are rarely described in aspirates.[33]

Other Causes of Lymphadenitis

Lymphadenopathy may occur in immunologic disorders such as systemic lupus erythematosus and rheuma-

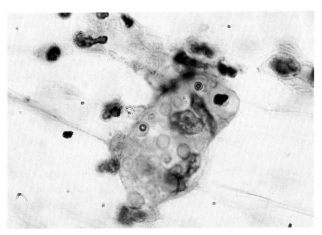
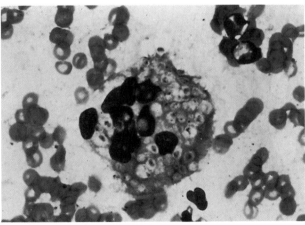

A   B

FIG. 4-8. Cryptococcal lymphadenitis. Observe budding giant cells containing organisms with surrounding capsule. The fungi usually have single buds, which are attached to the organism with a thin isthmus. (**A**, Papanicolaou stain, ×400; **B**, Diff-Quik stain, ×400. Courtesy of Yener S. Erozan, M.D., The Johns Hopkins University, Baltimore)

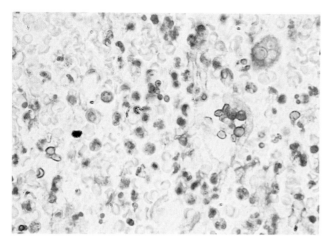

FIG. 4-9. Cryptococcal lymphadenitis. Capsule of the organism stains positively with mucin stains. (Mucicarmine stain, ×250)

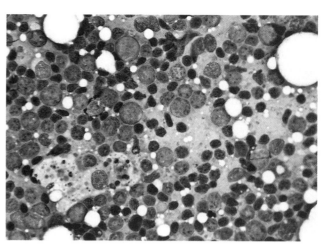

FIG. 4-11. Florid lymphoid hyperplasia. Transformed lymphocytes, paraimmunoblasts, and tingible body macrophages are present in a lymph node aspirate from a patient infected with HIV. (Diff-Quik stain, ×500)

toid arthritis. Drug-related lymphadenopathy may occur from hypersensitivity to phenytoin, particularly Dilantin; aspirates show prominent immunoblasts and rarely Reed-Sternberg–like cells. FNA biopsy has been shown to be helpful in cases of clinically suspected sarcoidosis.[34,35] Smears show epithelioid histiocytes without necrosis, multinucleated giant cells, and lymphocytes. Infectious etiologies should be excluded. Asteroid bodies and Schaumann bodies have been described in association with sarcoidosis, but these findings are nonspecific.[36]

LYMPHOMAS

Non-Hodgkin's Lymphoma

Diagnosing lymphoproliferative disorders by FNA is difficult mainly because of the lack of standardization of

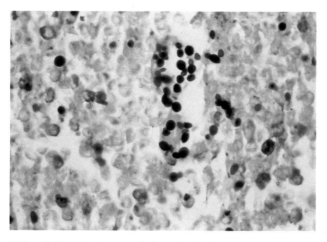

FIG. 4-10. Cryptococcal lymphadenitis. Budding yeast forms stain strongly with methenamine silver. (Methenamine silver stain, ×250)

terminology with regard to lymphoma classification by histology and cytology and the complexity of histologic categorization of many of the subtypes. A number of systems have been used to classify non-Hodgkin's lymphomas by histology. The Kiel classification developed by Lennert is used in Europe and has been recently updated.[37,38] It is based on the postulated relationship of neoplastic cells to their normal lymphoid counterparts, and specific entities are defined using morphologic and immunologic criteria. The Working Formulation developed by the National Cancer Institute is most widely used in the United States.[39] This classification is based on both on morphology and biologic behavior of lymphoma. It is divided into low-, intermediate-, and high-grade tumors. The morphologic features are further subdivided to indicate a diffuse or follicular growth pattern. This classification system is adaptable to cytologic specimens, but fewer categories exist in cytopathology because of the inability to assess the architectural features that differentiate follicular and diffuse subtypes.

An international group of hematopathologists has proposed a new revised European-American classification[40] based on a large number of distinct lymphomas that are defined using morphologic, immunophenotypic, genotypic, and clinical criteria (Table 4-1). This classification may well supplant the Kiel classification and the Working Formulation, which is based on hematoxylin-eosin–stained sections without the benefit of current immunologic or molecular genetic techniques. Many of the entities proposed include both nodal and extra-nodal lymphoma and are broadly grouped into three major categories of lymphoid malignancies, namely B-cell lymphoma, T-cell lymphoma, and Hodgkin's disease.

Although controversial, not all lymphoproliferative disorders diagnosed by FNA biopsy need subsequent his-

TABLE 4-1. *Revised European-American classification*

B-CELL NEOPLASMS

Precursor B-cell neoplasm: precursor B-lymphoblastic leukemia, lymphoma

Peripheral B-cell neoplasms

    B-cell chronic lymphocytic leukemia, prolymphocytic leukemia, small lymphocytic lymphoma

    Lymphoplasmacytoid lymphoma, immunocytoma

    Mantle cell lymphoma

    Follicle center lymphoma, follicular

        Provisional cytologic grades: I (small cell), II (mixed small and large cell), III (large cell)

        Provisional subtype: diffuse, predominantly small cell type

    Marginal zone B-cell lymphoma

        Extranodal (MALT-type with or without monocytoid B cells)

        Provisional subtype: nodal (with or without monocytoid B cells)

    Provisional entity: splenic marginal zone lymphoma (with or without villous lymphocytes)

    Hairy cell leukemia

    Plasmacytoma, plasma cell myeloma

    Diffuse large B-cell lymphoma*

        Subtype: primary mediastinal (thymic) B-cell lymphoma

    Burkitt's lymphoma

    Provisional entity: high-grade B-cell lymphoma, Burkitt's-like*

T-CELL AND PUTATIVE NATURAL KILLER CELL NEOPLASMS

Precursor T-cell neoplasm: precursor T-lymphoblastic lymphoma, leukemia

Peripheral T-cell and natural killer cell neoplasms

    T cell chronic lymphocytic leukemia, prolymphocytic leukemia

    Large granular lymphocyte leukemia

        T-cell type

        Natural killer cell type

    Mycosis fungoides, Sézary's syndrome

    Peripheral T-cell lymphomas, unspecified*

        Provisional cytologic categories: medium-sized cell, mixed medium and large cell, large cell, lymphoepithelioid cell

        Provisional subtype: hepatosplenic γδ T-cell lymphoma

        Provisional subtype: subcutaneous panniculitic T-cell lymphoma

    Angioimmunoblastic T-cell lymphoma

    Angiocentric lymphoma

    Intestinal T-cell lymphoma (enteropathy associated or not)

    Adult T-cell lymphoma, leukemia

    Anaplastic large cell lymphoma, CD30+, T- and null-cell types

    Provisional entity: anaplastic large cell lymphoma, Hodgkin's-like

HODGKIN'S DISEASE

Lymphocyte predominance

Nodular sclerosis

Mixed cellularity

Lymphocyte depletion

Provisional entity: lymphocyte-rich, classic Hodgkin's disease

---

MALT, mucosa-associated lymphoid tissue.

* These categories are thought likely to include more than one disease entity.

(Adapted from Harris NL, Jaffe ES, Stein H, et al. A revised European-American classification of lymphoid neoplasms: a proposal from the international lymphoma study group. Blood 1994;84:1361)

---

tologic confirmation. Certain lymphomas such as follicular center lymphoma, mantle cell lymphoma, marginal zone lymphoma, mucosa-associated lymphoid tissue (MALT) lymphoma, and Hodgkin's disease require histologic confirmation for an accurate initial diagnosis to assess the architectural pattern or to further subclassify the lymphoma, as in the case of Hodgkin's disease. How-ever, other disorders, such as reactive lymphoid hyperplasia, small lymphocytic lymphoma, large cell lymphoma, immunoblastic lymphoma, and anaplastic large cell Ki-1 positive lymphoma, do not require evaluation of the architecture. They have distinctive cytologic, immunophenotypic, and ploidy profiles, and therefore, a definitive diagnosis can be rendered on cytologic preparations.[3,15] T-cell lymphomas are usually more difficult to diagnose on cytologic preparations than are B-cell lymphomas because there is no immunophenotypic marker analogous to isotype light-chain restriction. A diagnosis of T-cell lymphoma requires the demonstration of T-cell antigens (CD3, CD4, CD5, and CD8) or T-cell subset antigen restriction in morphologically atypical cells. In some T-cell lymphomas there is loss of pan–T-cell antigens.[41]

The classification of lymphoma by FNA is based on a multiparameter approach combining the cytologic features using the modified Working Formulation (Table 4-2) with immunophenotyping, DNA ploidy analysis, and molecular studies when indicated. Pertinent clinical information such as age of patient, sites of involvement, and peripheral blood and bone marrow status is important in evaluating the case.[3] Accurate interpretation requires optimally prepared cytologic smears. Air-dried smears stained with Diff-Quik (Romanowsky stain) are helpful in assessing the cytoplasm and cell size relative to red blood cells. This stain is essential in evaluating lymphoproliferative disorders. Nuclear features, however, are better seen on alcohol-fixed, Papanicolaou-stained smears. Optimally, both air-dried and alcohol-fixed smears should be made because they are complementary.

A lymphoproliferative process, either benign or malignant, should be suspected when an aspirate shows a dispersed single-cell population of lymphoid cells with lymphoglandular bodies in the background. Lymphoglandular bodies are cytoplasmic fragments that stain green-gray on Papanicolaou stain and blue-gray with Diff-Quik. When evaluating a lymphoproliferative disorder, one should assess the cytologic features and cell composition. The cell size may be small (equal or slightly larger than a normal resting lymphocyte), intermediate (one and one-half times the size of a normal lymphocyte and no greater than the nucleus of a histiocyte), or large (two to three times the size of a normal lymphocyte). The nuclei may be round, indented, or cleaved or complex and lobulated. The cell composition may be monomorphous with one cell population predominating or polymorphous, containing a mixed population of different sized cells. Monomorphic lymphoid processes can be categorized into three groups on the basis of cell size: (1) small cells—small lymphocytic lymphoma, mantle cell lymphoma, and small cleaved cell lymphoma; (2) intermediate cells—small noncleaved cell or Burkitt's lymphoma and lymphoblastic lymphoma; (3) large cells—large cell lymphoma, immunoblastic lymphoma, and

TABLE 4-2. *Classification adopted from the working formulation for non-Hodgkin's lymphoma*

Histologic classification	Cytologic equivalent	Fine needle aspirate appearance
LOW GRADE		
Small lymphocytic, small lymphocytic plasmacytoid	Small lymphocytic, small lymphocytic plasmacytoid	
Mantle cell, mantle zone	Mantle cell	
Follicular small cleaved cell	Small cleaved cell	
Follicular small cleaved and large cell	Mixed small cleaved and large cell	
INTERMEDIATE GRADE		
Follicular large cell	Large cell	
Diffuse small cleaved cell, diffuse mantle cell	Small cleaved cell, mantle cell	
Diffuse mixed small cleaved and large cell	Mixed small cleaved and large cell	
Follicular large cell, diffuse large cell	Large cell	
HIGH GRADE		
Large cell, immunoblastic	Large cell, immunoblastic	
Lymphoblastic	Lymphoblastic	
Small noncleaved cell	Small noncleaved cell	

(Adapted from Katz RL, Wojcik EM, Johnston DA. Image analysis in non-Hodgkin's lymphoma emphasizing applications in tissue procured by fine needle aspiration. In: Wied GL, Bartels PH, et al., eds. Compendium on the computerized cytology and histology. St. Louis, MO, Science Printers and Publishers, 1993)

granulocytic sarcoma. Polymorphic lymphoid processes include reactive hyperplasia, mixed cell lymphoma, Hodgkin's disease, and monomorphic processes admixed with nonneoplastic lymphoid tissue.[3] The latter may be due to partial involvement of a lymph node by lymphoma or peripheral blood contamination with T lymphocytes.

Determination of monoclonality confirms the diagnosis of lymphoma. To demonstrate monoclonality by immunophenotyping on cytospin preparations, it is necessary to use a panel of antibodies to the light-chain immunoglobulins, kappa and lambda, and a pan–T-cell antigen (CD3). If small lymphocytic, mantle cell, or marginal zone lymphoma is suspected, CD5 (a pan–T-cell an-

tigen that is also expressed on a minor subset of B lymphocytes) is also included. A monoclonal population demonstrating light-chain restriction is defined as a kappa/lambda ratio of 6:1 or more or lambda/kappa ratio of 4:1 or more. Most lymphomas show monotypic staining in 80% to 90% of the neoplastic cells.[8] Polyclonal populations show a mixture of cells staining for kappa, lambda, and CD3. The kappa/lambda ratio should not exceed 3:1, and the lambda/kappa ratio should not exceed 2:1. When the light-chain expression is intermediate between the definition of monoclonality and polyclonality, it is regarded as inconclusive for monoclonality, and an excisional biopsy is necessary for a definitive diagnosis. This may occur when there is partial involvement of a lymph node by lymphoma or atypical lymphoid hyperplasia.[3]

An important aid to diagnosing lymphomas by FNA has been the development of instrumentation, either flow cytometry or image analysis systems, that can quantitate DNA content throughout the cell cycle and produce a distinctive histogram pattern according to the grade of lymphoma. In addition, antibodies against proliferation markers, notably Ki-67, may be used to supplement or substitute for kinetic studies. Flow cytometry provides a rapid and quantitative method for measuring various phases of the cell cycle. At our institution, acridine orange, a dye that binds stoichiometrically with DNA and RNA content, has been used for flow cytometry measurements in lymphomas derived from excised lymph nodes and FNA biopsies. The flow cytometric analysis of DNA ploidy, RNA content, and proliferative activity (S+G2M%) has been shown to correlate with the grade of the lymphoma when using the Working Formulation.[10,42] As the grade of lymphoma increases, there is a progressive increase in the RNA content and proliferative activity. Lymphomas are subdivided on the basis of the percentage of cells in the proliferative phase (S+G2M%) into low (less than 5%), intermediate (5% to 15%), and high (more than 15%) grades. More recently, ploidy determination by DNA image analysis was shown to have a strong correlation with the grade and outcome of lymphoma.[42,43] Ploidy analysis is particularly useful in aspirates that yield low cellularity and can be performed on a single cytospin preparation prepared in a similar manner as for immunocytochemical analysis. By image analysis (SAMBA 4000 cell analyzer, Image Products International, Inc, Chantilly, VA), six different histogram patterns have been defined based on proliferation index and cells with DNA content greater than 5 c. Low-grade lymphomas are usually diploid with a proliferation index less than 1.2 with or without cells with DNA content greater than 5 c; intermediate-grade lymphomas are diploid or aneuploid with a proliferation index between 1.2 and 4.0 with or without cells with DNA content greater than 5 c. High-grade lymphomas are mostly diploid, except for Ki-1 positive large cell anaplastic type and have a proliferation index of more than 4.0 with or without cells with DNA content greater than 5 c.[42] Ki-67 is an antibody that detects cells in the early G1 phase and throughout the cell cycle. Katz and colleagues[42] and Erler and Katz[44] demonstrated that Ki-67 performed on a single cytospin preparation correlates with the grade and subtype of lymphoma by the Working Formulation. A cutoff of 26% is used to separate low-grade versus high-grade lymphomas.

Low-Grade Lymphoma

Small Lymphocytic Lymphoma

Small lymphocytic lymphoma occurs in late adult life, peaking in the sixth or seventh decade. It usually presents with generalized lymphadenopathy and bone marrow involvement.

Cytopathology. Aspirates are usually hypercellular and consist of a monotonous population of small, mature, round lymphocytes. Nuclei are smaller than histiocyte nuclei and have coarsely clumped "checkerboard" chromatin (Fig. 4-12). Small nucleoli may or may not be identified. Scattered among the small lymphocytes are a subpopulation of larger lymphoid cells, namely, paraimmunoblasts (Fig. 4-13) and prolymphocytes, which have abundant pale cytoplasm, fine nuclear chromatin, and central nucleoli. These cells represent the pseudofollicles or proliferation centers seen on histologic sections. Mitoses are rarely identified. Chronic lymphocytic leukemia, the leukemic counterpart of small lymphocytic lymphoma, shows identical cytomorphology.

In the accelerated phase of small lymphocytic lymphoma, the morphology is similar but increased numbers of mitotic figures are present. Transformation to large cell lymphoma (Richter's syndrome) or immunoblastic sarcoma occurs in about 10% to 15% of cases.[45]

Ancillary Studies. Most small lymphocytic lymphomas are B-cell neoplasms and express one of the surface immunoglobulin (sIg) light chains (kappa or lambda) (Fig. 4-14), IgM (faint staining), occasionally IgD, B-cell–associated antigens (CD19, CD20), CD5, and CD23. An important differentiating feature is that most small lymphocytic lymphomas are positive for CD5 and negative for CD10 (common acute lymphocytic leukemia antigen). Rare cases demonstrate T-cell markers consistent with peripheral T-cell lymphoma.

Cytokinetic studies show a diploid population with low RNA content and low proliferative activity. Ki-67 expression is low with a mean value of less than 10%.[19] Transformed lymphomas (Richter's syndrome) are characterized by increased proliferative activity, and the Ki-67 activity is usually greater than 26%.

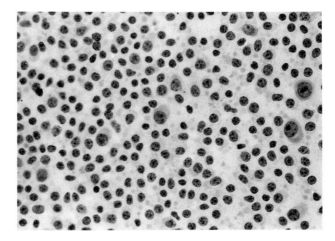

FIG. 4-12. Small lymphocytic lymphoma. Smear is composed predominantly of small round lymphocytes with a checkerboard chromatin pattern and rare paraimmunoblasts. (Papanicolaou stain, ×500)

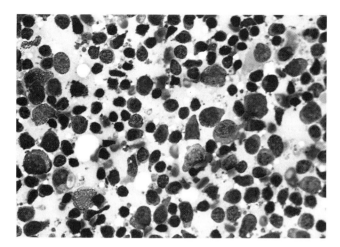

FIG. 4-13. Small lymphocytic lymphoma. Lymph node aspirate shows small mature lymphocytes with an increased number of paraimmunoblasts. (Diff-Quik stain, ×500)

Differential Diagnosis. Reactive hyperplasia, medullary cord expansion, Castleman's disease, and small cleaved cell lymphoma are diagnostic considerations. Most of these entities can be differentiated with confidence using immunophenotyping. Benign processes are polyclonal and show a polymorphous population of lymphocytes, plasma cells, and histiocytes. Small lymphocytic lymphoma differs from mantle cell lymphoma in possessing smaller rounder nuclei with coarser chromatin. Although these two entities may be similar immunophenotypically, only small lymphocytic lymphoma is CD23 positive.[46]

Small Lymphocytic Lymphoma, Plasmacytoid

Small lymphocytic plasmacytoid lymphoma shows a similar age distribution as small lymphocytic lymphoma. Clinically this disease often presents with localized lymph node disease, but occasionally it also involves the spleen, orbit, salivary gland, lung, or gastrointestinal tract. It may be associated with hyperviscosity syndrome (Waldenström's macroglobulinemia) caused by severe paraproteinemia.

Cytopathology. Smears are composed of plasmacytoid lymphocytes, small mature lymphocytes, and occasional plasma cells. Plasmacytoid lymphocytes have abundant cytoplasm, eccentrically located nuclei, and diffuse nuclear chromatin similar to small lymphocytes. The typical "cartwheel" nuclear pattern and paranuclear clear zone seen in plasma cells is absent.

Ancillary Studies. The cells usually secrete sIg light chains kappa or lambda and IgM but are IgD negative. They usually are positive for pan–B-cell antigens (CD19, CD20) and lack CD10 and CD5.

Cytokinetic studies usually show a diploid population with an elevated RNA content, but proliferative activity is low. Ki-67 expression is low with a mean value of 12%.[44]

Differential Diagnosis. Small lymphocytic lymphoma, benign lymphoid proliferation (Castleman's disease, plasma cell variant), and plasmacytoma are diagnostic considerations. The plasmacytoid appearance of the cells, strong cytoplasmic sIg staining, and frequent lack of CD5 positivity are helpful in distinguishing small lymphocytic plasmacytoid lymphoma from small lymphocytic lymphoma. A polyclonal population would distinguish benign processes. Plasmacytomas are usually positive for IgG or IgA and are aneuploid, with a very high RNA content and proliferative activity. In contrast to plasmacytoma, bone marrow is not the site of plasmacytoid lymphomas, and therefore, clinical and radiographic findings are helpful.

Mantle Cell Lymphoma

Mantle cell lymphoma, previously known as intermediate cell lymphoma or centrocytic lymphoma, occurs in late adult life and is uncommon in individuals under 50 years of age. Generalized lymphadenopathy is the common presentation. The underlying histologic pattern may be mantle zone, wherein a wide mantle of small atypical cells surrounds normal or reactive germinal centers or may have a diffuse pattern with obliteration of normal lymph node architecture.

Cytopathology. Smears are composed exclusively of small- to medium-sized lymphocytes, usually slightly larger than normal lymphocytes. In most cases the nuclei are irregular, cleaved, or indented, but they may also be round, resembling small lymphocytes (Figs. 4-15 and 4-16). The chromatin pattern is less coarse than that seen in small lymphocytic lymphoma. Nucleoli are small and

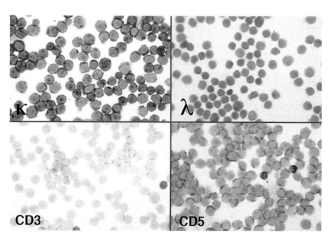

FIG. 4-14. Small lymphocytic lymphoma. Immunocytochemical studies show the following positive percentages: kappa 98%, lambda 1%, CD3 1%, and CD5 90%. Note CD5 staining is faint in B cells compared with that in T cells. (Immunoperoxidase stain, ×500)

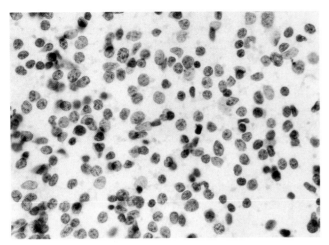

FIG. 4-15. Mantle cell lymphoma. Lymph node aspirate shows intermediate-sized cells with round or cleaved nuclei. (Papanicolaou stain, ×500)

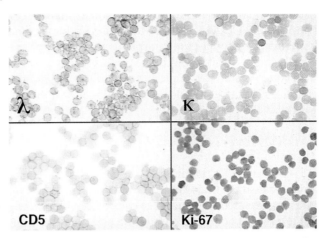

FIG. 4-17. Mantle cell lymphoma. Immunostaining shows the following positive percentages: lambda 70%, kappa 5%, CD3 95%, and Ki-67 50%. (Immunoperoxidase stain, ×500)

inconspicuous. Transformed cells (paraimmunoblasts or centroblasts) are extremely rare or absent. Mitoses vary from zero to two per high-power field; greater than two mitoses per high-power field have been observed in those corresponding to larger cell types. A lymphoblastic variant composed of intermediate-sized cells, resembling lymphoblasts of lymphoblastic lymphoma, exists. This may show variable numbers of tingible body macrophages and increased number of mitoses and is associated with a shorter survival time.[47]

Ancillary Studies. Cells have an immature monoclonal B-cell phenotype expressing sIgM and frequently IgD. Lambda–light-chain restriction is more common than kappa–light-chain restriction (Fig. 4-17). They stain positively for pan–B-cell antigens (CD19, CD20, CD22, and CD24) and CD5, and variably for CD10.

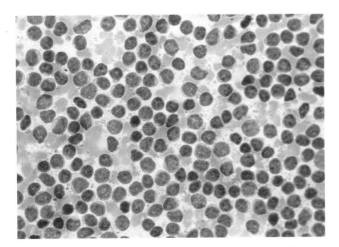

FIG. 4-16. Mantle cell lymphoma. Air-dried smears show a monomorphous population of cells. Note the absence of paraimmunoblasts. (Diff-Quik stain, ×500)

Cytokinetic studies usually show a diploid population with low RNA content and low to intermediate proliferative activity. The intermediate-grade tumors often show frequent mitoses and increased expression of Ki-67 antigen and have a more aggressive clinical course.[43]

Molecular studies show that most tumor cells have a chromosomal translocation t(11;14) that involves the *bcl*-1 locus on the long arm of chromosome 11. This translocation results in the overexpression of a gene called *PRAD* 1, which encodes a cyclin product that is thought to abrogate normal cell cycle checkpoints, resulting in the unregulated proliferation of neoplastic cells.[11]

Differential Diagnosis. Lymphoblastic lymphoma, small lymphocytic lymphoma, small cleaved cell lymphoma, mixed small and large cell lymphoma, and marginal zone lymphoma (monocytoid B-cell lymphoma or MALT lymphoma) are diagnostic considerations. Difficulty may occur in separating mantle cell lymphoma from lymphoblastic lymphoma because both have light staining irregular nuclei; however, the cytoplasm of lymphoblastic lymphoma is basophilic compared with the grayish cytoplasm of mantle cell lymphoma on air-dried smears stained with Diff-Quik or other Romanowsky stains. A high mitotic activity and younger age group of patients favors lymphoblastic lymphoma. Immunophenotyping can distinguish these two entities because lymphoblastic lymphoma usually demonstrates cortical thymic markers (CD1, CD2, CD3, CD4, CD5, and CD8) or pre–B-cell markers (CD10, CD19, and CD20), as well as terminal deoxynucleotidyl transferase (TdT). The presence of a monomorphic population and the absence of paraimmunoblasts is helpful in differentiating small lymphocytic lymphoma, small cleaved cell lymphoma, and mixed small cleaved and large cell lymphoma from mantle cell lymphoma. In contrast to small lymphocytic lymphoma, mantle cell lymphoma is CD23 negative. Marginal zone lymphoma is characterized by a monomorphous to polymorphous population of small round to cleaved (centrocytic) cells with variable numbers of plasma cells; it is characteristically CD5 negative as opposed to mantle cell lymphoma, which is CD5 positive.

Follicular Center Lymphoma

Follicular center lymphomas are of B-cell lineage and are subclassified into small cleaved cell, mixed small cleaved and large cell, and large cleaved cell lymphoma but are actually part of a continuum based on the number of large noncleaved cells (centroblasts). Classification on cytologic specimens is further complicated by the admixture of interfollicular T cells; however, if immunophenotyping is performed these cells could be excluded from the grading system.

No cytologically defined criteria separate these entities. With new patients, we advocate excisional biopsy to classify these follicular center lymphomas further. We use an arbitrary cytologic classification loosely based on the histologic criteria of Mann and Berard[48]: (1) small cleaved cell lymphoma—small cleaved cells with less than 5% large noncleaved cells per high-power field, (2) mixed small cleaved and large cell lymphoma—small cleaved cells are admixed with a significant component of large cleaved cells and 5% to 10% of large noncleaved cells per high-power field, and (3) large cleaved cell lymphoma—predominance of large cleaved cells or greater than 10% large noncleaved cells per high-power field. We would point out, however, that even histologic criteria for classification of these subtypes of follicular center lymphomas are controversial. Recently a group of international hematopathologists[11] proposed grading follicular center lymphomas from one to three on the basis of Mann and Berard criteria. A grading system should have prognostic and therapeutic implications. It has been shown that using Mann and Berard criteria for diagnosis, patients with small cleaved cell type continue to relapse at a steady rate, whereas patients diagnosed with mixed small cleaved and large cell lymphoma may have complete remission with combination chemotherapy. According to the Working Formulation small cleaved cell lymphoma and mixed small cleaved and large cell lymphomas are low-grade lymphomas, whereas large cleaved cell lymphoma is classified as an intermediate-grade lymphoma. This latter point is questionable, because the relapse pattern of large cleaved cell lymphoma after therapy tends to show a steady rate similar to that of low-grade follicular center lymphomas. It is recommended that each institution formulate its own set of criteria to grade these follicular center lymphomas until data from prospective clinical trials are available to suggest a uniform method.[40]

Cytopathology. Small cleaved cell lymphoma is composed primarily of small cells slightly larger than mature lymphocytes with scant cytoplasm, moderately to markedly irregular or "twisted" nuclear contours, and small nucleoli (Fig. 4-18). Less than 5% of the population is composed of large noncleaved cells, which are characterized by large round nuclei with fine chromatin and two to three peripherally placed nucleoli.

Mixed cell lymphoma is composed of small and large cleaved cells and between 5% and 10% of large noncleaved cells. Small cleaved cells and large cells should be present in equal numbers to make the diagnosis (Figs. 4-19 and 4-20).

Large cell lymphoma has large cells with irregular nuclear contours, vesicular chromatin, inconspicuous nucleoli, and scant cytoplasm, as well as variable numbers of large noncleaved cells, ranging from 10% upward (Figs. 4-21 and 4-22).

Ancillary Studies. Follicular center lymphomas are of B-cell lineage and show monotypic staining for either kappa or lambda sIg, and IgM, IgG, or IgA. They are usually CD5 negative, variably CD10 positive, and express pan–B-cell markers (CD19, CD20, CD22). There may be numerous T cells representing the interfollicular cells; counts up to 40% have been reported.

On tissue sections, *bcl*-2 protein expression has been shown to be useful in distinguishing reactive from neoplastic follicles, because it is absent in the former and present in most follicular lymphomas.[49,50] In cytologic preparations, however, it is not helpful because interfollicular T cells also express this antigen.

Cytokinetic studies of small cleaved cell lymphoma show a diploid population with low RNA content and proliferative activity. Ki-67 expression is low (less than 10%) and is seen primarily in the large noncleaved (centroblast) cells. Mixed small cleaved and large cell

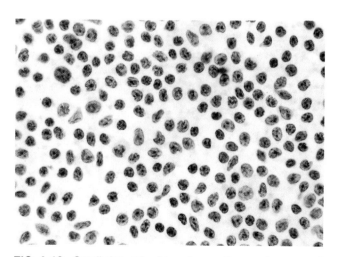

FIG. 4-18. Small cleaved cell lymphoma. Smear shows small cells with markedly irregular nuclei and rare large noncleaved cells. (Papanicolaou stain, ×500)

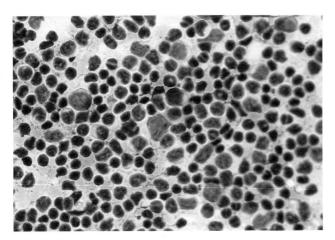

FIG. 4-19. Mixed small cleaved and large cell lymphoma. Lymph node aspirate is composed of an admixture of small and large cleaved cells and large noncleaved cells. (Diff-Quik stain, ×500)

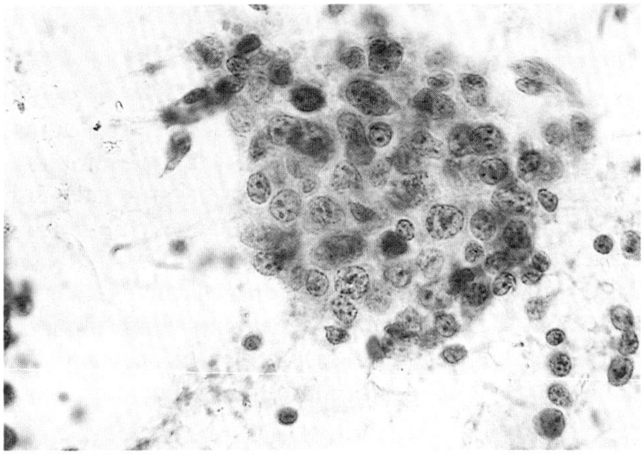

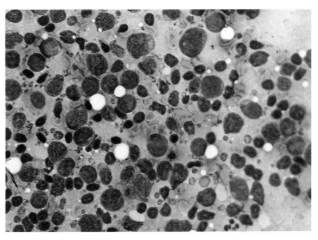

FIG. 4-21. Large cell lymphoma. Lymph node aspirate shows an aggregate of large noncleaved cells derived from a follicular center lymphoma. (Papanicolaou stain, ×500)

lymphoma shows a diploid population that sometimes coexists with a smaller aneuploid subpopulation and has a low proliferative activity. About 15% of malignant cells express Ki-67 positivity. Large cell lymphoma shows a predominant diploid or aneuploid subpopulation with an intermediate proliferative activity. Ki-67 is usually positive in about 20% to 25% of cells.

Cytogenetic studies reveal that 70% to 80% of follicular center lymphomas have the (14;18) chromosomal translocation involving the rearrangement of the *bcl-2* gene, which results in the expression of *bcl-2* protein believed to immortalize the neoplastic B cells.[40]

Differential Diagnosis. Reactive hyperplasia, small lymphocytic lymphoma, and mantle cell lymphoma are diagnostic considerations in cases of small cleaved cell lymphoma. Reactive hyperplasia shows a polyclonal

polymorphous lymphoid population along with tingible body macrophages, plasma cells, and histiocytes. Small lymphocytic lymphoma shows small round lymphocytes with coarsely clumped chromatin. Both small lymphocytic lymphoma and mantle cell lymphoma are CD5 positive in contrast to small cleaved cell lymphoma, which is CD5 negative.

In mixed small cleaved and large cell lymphoma and large cell lymphoma, the differential diagnosis includes mixed cell lymphoma of T-cell lineage (peripheral T-cell lymphoma) and reactive hyperplasia with increased immunoblasts, as discussed previously. Immunophenotyping is helpful in distinguishing follicular center (B-cell) lymphomas from T-cell lymphomas.

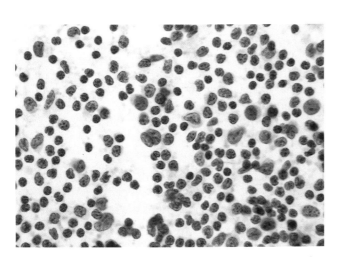

FIG. 4-20. Mixed small cleaved and large cell lymphoma. Observe the approximately equal numbers of small cleaved and large cells. (Papanicolaou stain, ×500)

FIG. 4-22. Large cell lymphoma, B-cell type. Aspirate consists primarily of large atypical lymphocytes with a few smaller lymphocytes that proved to be T cells by immunophenotyping. Note the presence of lymphoglandular bodies in the background. (Diff-Quik stain, ×500)

High-Grade Lymphoma

Large Cell Lymphoma

The high-grade large B-cell lymphomas have a diffuse growth pattern and account for 30% to 40% of adult non-Hodgkin's lymphomas. They usually occur in late adult life, but the age range is broad and includes children and adolescents. Patients typically present with a rapidly enlarging mass. Although these neoplasms are biologically aggressive, they are potentially curable with multiagent high-dose chemotherapy. Included in this category are diffuse large noncleaved cell, multilobated, and immunoblastic lymphomas.

Cytopathology. The cells are large and have nuclei that are at least twice the size of a small lymphocyte and usually larger than histocyte nuclei. Nuclei have vesicular chromatin and one or more nucleoli (Fig. 4-23). A distinct rim of cytoplasm is present that may be vacuolated. The neoplastic cells resemble centroblasts (large noncleaved cells). Immunoblastic lymphomas are usually characterized by a monomorphous population of large cells with large eccentrically placed nuclei, prominent centrally placed nuclei, paranuclear clearing, and basophilic cytoplasm (Fig. 4-24). Multilobated B-cell lymphoma has large irregular nuclei with bulbous protrusions and concavities. Some cases may contain numerous small T lymphocytes or histiocytes.

Ancillary Studies. Tumor cells are positive for pan–B-cell markers (CD19, CD20, CD22) and show variable staining for CD5 and CD10. They may or may not show sIg.

Cytokinetic studies usually show a diploid population, a high RNA content, and a very high proliferative activity. Ki-67 expression is high (more than 50%).

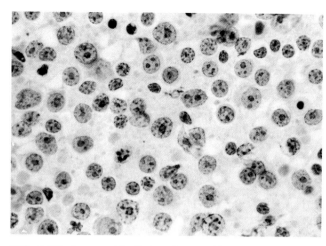

FIG. 4-24. Immunoblastic lymphoma. Observe the eccentrically placed, large, round nuclei with prominent central nucleoli. (Papanicolaou stain, ×500)

Differential Diagnosis. Reactive hyperplasia with immunoblasts, granulocytic sarcoma, plasmacytoma, melanoma, nasopharyngeal carcinoma, and seminoma are diagnostic considerations. Large cell lymphoma may be difficult to distinguish from reactive hyperplasia with increased numbers of immunoblasts by cytomorphology alone; however, reactive nodes usually show a polyclonal immunophenotype. Flow cytometry may be helpful. Although both large cell lymphoma and reactive hyperplasia may show elevated proliferative activity, a certain percentage of large cell lymphomas are aneuploid. Aspirates of granulocytic sarcoma (chloroma) may be composed primarily of blasts with round to oval nuclei and basophilic cytoplasm. Some cases are agranular, and others contain granules that are best seen on Diff-Quik preparations. Granules that stain positively for Naphthol AS-D chloroacetate (NASD) and myeloperoxidase are helpful in differentiating granulocytic sarcoma from large cell lymphoma.[3] Plasmacytoma (Fig. 4-25) is usually IgA or IgG positive. Clinical and radiographic data may be helpful in separating these two entities. Melanoma is positive for melanin antigen, HMB-45, and S-100 protein. Undifferentiated carcinoma, particularly nasopharyngeal carcinoma, may be cytologically similar to lymphoma. The presence of cohesive epithelial groups and positive immunostaining for keratin supports a diagnosis of carcinoma.

Anaplastic Large Cell Lymphoma (Ki-1 Positive)

Anaplastic large cell lymphoma is a rare neoplasm that has been reported in all age groups. Although most cases arise de novo, some patients have a history of another type of lymphoma. Two distinct forms of anaplastic large cell lymphoma exist, systemic and cutaneous. The systemic form, which may involve lymph nodes or extra-

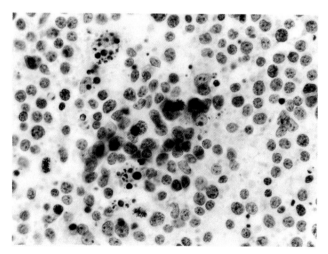

FIG. 4-23. High-grade large cell lymphoma. Most of the cells are large and noncleaved with a high mitotic rate. The presence of tingible body macrophages is not always indicative of a benign process. (Papanicolaou stain, ×500)

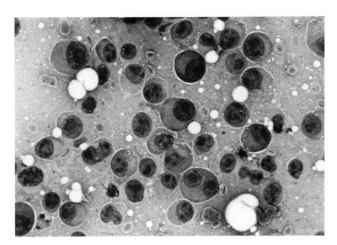

FIG. 4-25. Plasmacytoma. Aspirate shows a dispersed population of cells with abundant basophilic cytoplasm, eccentrically located nuclei, and prominent nucleoli. (Diff-Quik stain, ×500)

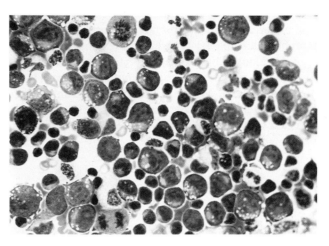

FIG. 4-27. Anaplastic large cell lymphoma. Cytospin preparation shows large cells with basophilic vacuolated cytoplasm. The cells are fairly uniform, consistent with the monomorphic variant of anaplastic large cell lymphoma. (Diff-Quik stain, ×500)

nodal sites, has a bimodal age distribution in children and adults and is clinically more aggressive. The primary cutaneous form occurs mostly in adults and can regress spontaneously. The term *anaplastic large cell lymphoma Hodgkin's-like* has been proposed for a tumor that is composed of cells similar to classic anaplastic large cell lymphoma but has architectural features that resemble nodular sclerosing Hodgkin's disease. This tumor usually occurs in the mediastinum of young adults and does not respond well to conventional therapy for Hodgkin's disease.[40]

Cytopathology. The tumor is composed of large cells with varying degrees of pleomorphism. Cells are often horseshoe-shaped or have multiple nuclei with multiple or single prominent nucleoli. Binucleated cells resembling Reed-Sternberg cells may be observed (Fig. 4-26). Tumor cells have abundant cytoplasm often vacuolated

(Fig. 4-27) and are much larger than the usual large cell lymphoma. A lymphohistiocytic and small cell variant of anaplastic large cell lymphoma have also been described.

Ancillary Studies. Anaplastic lymphomas characteristically show strong paranuclear or golgi-like positivity for Ki-1 (CD30) antibody (Fig. 4-28). Epithelial membrane antigen is positive in the systemic form but not in the primary cutaneous tumors. Most of these lymphomas are of T-cell origin with only a few having a B-cell or null-cell phenotype. Some are negative for T- and B-cell markers and negative or weakly positive for the leukocyte common antigen (LCA).

Cytokinetic studies show a diploid or aneuploid population with high proliferative activity. Ki-67 expression is high (more than 26%).

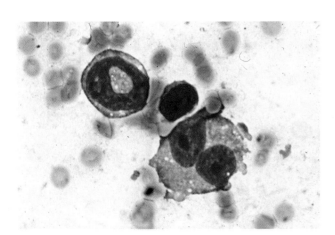

FIG. 4-26. Anaplastic large cell lymphoma. Large pleomorphic cells, one resembling a Reed-Sternberg cell and the other having a horseshoe-shaped nucleus, are present in a cervical lymph node aspirate. (Diff-Quik stain, ×1000)

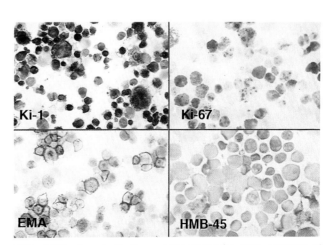

FIG. 4-28. Anaplastic large cell lymphoma. The majority of cells show positive immunostaining for Ki-1, Ki-67, and epithelial membrane antigen but show negative staining for HMB-45. (Immunoperoxidase stain, ×500)

Differential Diagnosis. Metastatic carcinoma, melanoma, sarcoma, malignant fibrous histiocytoma, and lymphocytic-depleted Hodgkin's disease are diagnostic considerations. Clinical history, cytologic features, and immunocytochemical studies including keratin, HMB-45, LCA, and Leu-M1 are helpful in distinguishing these entities. Hodgkin's disease, particularly the lymphocytic-depleted subtype, may be difficult to separate from anaplastic large cell lymphoma.

Small Noncleaved Cell Lymphoma

Small noncleaved cell lymphoma includes Burkitt's and Burkitt's-like (non-Burkitt's) lymphoma. Burkitt's lymphoma most commonly occurs in children. African (endemic) cases typically involve the face and jaw, whereas the non-African (nonendemic) cases often present in the abdomen and involve the distal ileum, cecum, and mesentery. Rare cases present as an acute leukemia and are subclassified as L3-ALL. The small noncleaved cell, Burkitt's-like type, may be seen in adults and is often associated with immunodeficiency.

Cytopathology. In Burkitt's lymphoma, smears are composed of medium-sized cells with uniform round nuclei and poorly preserved cytoplasm (Fig. 4-29). On Diff-Quik preparations, the cytoplasm is basophilic and contains small cytoplasmic vacuoles (Fig. 4-30). Nuclei have coarse chromatin and contain two to five distinct nucleoli. A "starry sky pattern" may be present as a result of an admixture of large tingible body macrophages (Fig. 4-31). Necrotic debris and mitotic figures are frequently present. The Burkitt's-like variant generally lacks the monotony seen in classic Burkitt's lymphoma; nuclei show moderate variation in size and shape and occasionally have a single prominent nucleoli.

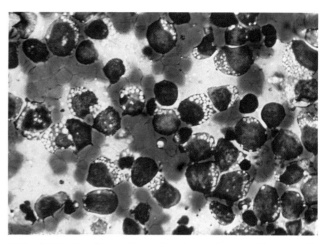

FIG. 4-30. Small noncleaved cell lymphoma. Tumor cells have basophilic cytoplasm containing multiple small vacuoles. (Diff-Quik stain, ×1000)

Ancillary Studies. Cells may or may not show light-chain restriction (Fig. 4-32). They are usually positive for pan–B-cell antigens (CD19, CD20, CD22), variably positive for CD10, and negative for CD5.

Cytokinetic studies usually show a diploid population, a high RNA content, and an extremely high proliferative activity. Ki-67 expression is high, about 80% to 90%.

Cytogenetic studies show reciprocal translocation involving chromosomes 8 and 14 in most cases.[40]

Differential Diagnosis. Small round cell tumors of childhood, melanoma, and lymphoblastic lymphoma are diagnostic considerations. In young patients, small noncleaved cell lymphoma must be differentiated from small round cell tumors of childhood and melanoma even though the latter is uncommon in children. The clinical presentation in conjunction with ancillary studies such as immunocytochemistry (desmin, muscle-

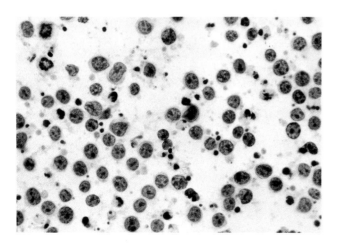

FIG. 4-29. Small noncleaved cell lymphoma (Burkitt's lymphoma). Lymph node aspirate shows intermediate-sized cells with round nuclei and two to three nucleoli. Observe the presence of cellular debris in the background. (Papanicolaou stain, ×500)

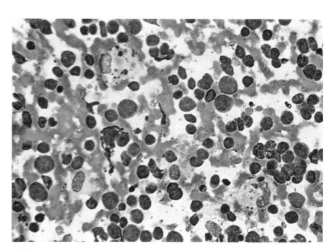

FIG. 4-31. Small noncleaved cell lymphoma. Tumor cells are admixed with tingible body macrophages. (Diff-Quik stain, ×400)

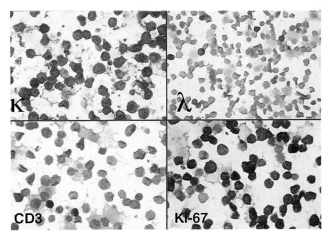

FIG. 4-32. Small noncleaved cell lymphoma. Immunocyto-chemical studies show the following positive percentages: kappa 95%, lambda 3%, CD3 2%, and Ki-67 85%. (Immuno-peroxidase stain, ×500)

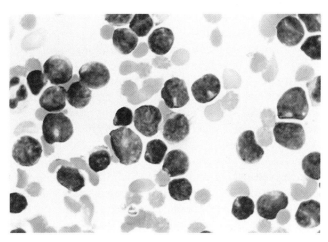

FIG. 4-34. Lymphoblastic lymphoma. High magnification shows a fine nuclear chromatin pattern and irregular nuclear outlines. Nucleoli are not prominent. (Diff-Quik stain, ×1000)

specific actin, neuron-specific enolase, and HMB-45) and ultrastructural analysis are helpful in distinguishing these entities without an open biopsy. Lymphoblastic lymphomas can be distinguished by their distinctive cytologic features (vide infra), distinctive clinical presentation (mediastinal mass with or without cervical lymph node involvement), predominantly immature T-cell phenotype, and TdT expression.

Lymphoblastic Lymphoma

Lymphoblastic lymphoma occurs in adolescents and young adults, primarily men, and presents as a rapidly enlarging mass, frequently involving the mediastinum. It is a neoplastic proliferation of transformed thymocytes and usually is of T-cell origin.

Cytopathology. Smears show a monomorphous pop-ulation of intermediate-sized cells that are slightly larger than small lymphocytes but smaller than cells of large cell lymphoma. Nuclei are lobulated and convoluted with infoldings of the nuclear membrane or round to oval (Figs. 4-33 and 4-34). They have fine chromatin and inconspicuous nucleoli. Cytoplasm is scant, basophilic, and nonvacuolated. Mitotic figures may be numerous. There is no correlation between cytomorphology and T- or B-cell lineage.

Ancillary Studies. Most lymphoblastic lymphomas are of T-cell lineage and have variable phenotypic mark-ers (Fig. 4-35). consistent with a cortical thymocyte phe-notype (CD1, CD2, CD3, CD4, CD5); CD4 and CD8 may be coexpressed. TdT is characteristically positive and is the most useful diagnostic marker. About 30% of these tumors express pan–B-cell markers (CD19, CD20)

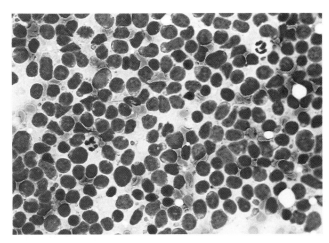

FIG. 4-33. Lymphoblastic lymphoma. Lymph node aspirate shows monotonous population of blastic cells with round nu-clei. (Diff-Quik stain, ×500)

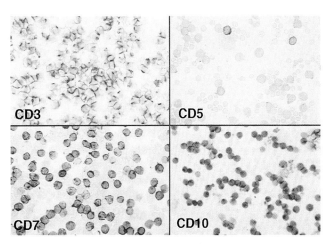

FIG. 4-35. Lymphoblastic lymphoma. Immunocytochemical studies show the following positive percentages: CD3 85%, CD5 75% (faint staining), CD7 90%, and CD10 85%. (Immu-noperoxidase stain, ×500)

and CD10. Rarely, a T-cell phenotype may coexist with myeloid differentiation.

Cytokinetic studies usually show a diploid population, a low RNA content, and an intermediate proliferative activity. Ki-67 expression is high (more than 26%).

Molecular studies usually show rearrangement in the Ig heavy chain (lineage infidelity), whereas rearrangement of T-cell receptor genes is present in only a minority of cases.[40]

Differential Diagnosis. Granulocytic sarcoma, small noncleaved cell lymphoma, and thymoma are diagnostic considerations. Granulocytic sarcoma may be distinguished by histochemical stains such as NASD, myeloperoxidase, and Sudan Black. Small noncleaved cell lymphoma and lymphoblastic lymphoma differ cytomorphologically, and the former is TdT negative.

Aspirates from the mediastinum should be interpreted with caution because lymphocytes from a thymoma may show a similar phenotype. However, the cytomorphologic features of the mature lymphocytes in a thymoma differ from the characteristic blastic morphology seen in lymphoblastic lymphoma.[51]

Peripheral T-Cell Lymphoma

Peripheral T-cell lymphoma comprises a heterogeneous but distinct group of postthymic lymphomas exclusive of mycosis fungoides, Sézary's syndrome, T-cell lymphoblastic lymphoma, and adult T-cell lymphoma/ leukemia. These tumors are often difficult to classify using the National Cancer Institute's Working Formulation.[52] This is due in part to the variation in cell size and nuclear irregularity along with the frequent admixture of "normal" cellular components such as epithelioid histiocytes, mature lymphocytes, and eosinophils. This difficulty in classification is particularly true of low-grade tu-

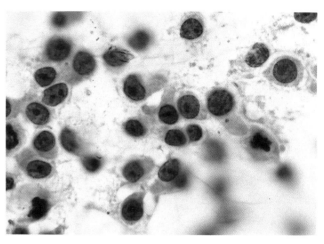

FIG. 4-37. High-grade T-cell lymphoma. Smear shows large cells with vesicular chromatin and prominent nucleoli. (Papanicolaou stain, ×1000)

mors that do not conform to the small lymphocytic or follicular small cleaved cell category in the Working Formulation.

Cytopathology. Smears may contain a variable combination of atypical small, intermediate, and large lymphoid cells (Figs. 4-36 and 4-37). The cells often have irregular nuclei that can vary considerably in size and shape. Occasional atypical mononucleated or binucleated cells resembling Reed-Sternberg cells have been reported. Epithelioid histiocytes and eosinophils may be numerous.

Ancillary Studies. Immunophenotyping is characterized by a predominance of T cells usually more than 70% to 80% of the cell population. Tumor cells show variable staining for T cell-associated antigens (CD2, CD3, CD5, CD7) (Fig. 4-38). Positivity for helper cells (CD4) frequently predominates over expression of suppressor cells

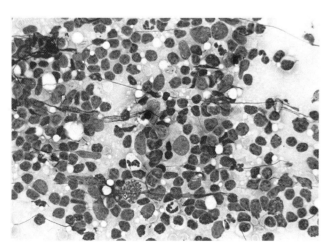

FIG. 4-36. T-cell lymphoma. Lymph node aspirate shows a mixed population of small and large atypical lymphoid cells. (Diff-Quik stain, ×400)

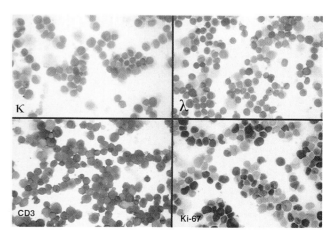

FIG. 4-38. High-grade T-cell lymphoma. Immunocytochemical studies show the following positive percentages: kappa 5%, lambda 5%, CD3 90%, and Ki-67 70%. (Immunoperoxidase stain, ×500)

(CD8). Other phenotypic aberrations such as loss of pan–T-cell antigens or coexpression of helper and suppressor phenotypes may occur. B cell-associated antigens are lacking.

Cytokinetic studies usually show a diploid population with intermediate proliferative activity.

Differential Diagnosis. Reactive hyperplasia and Hodgkin's lymphoma are diagnostic considerations. Peripheral T-cell lymphomas may be misinterpreted as a reactive process because of the frequent occurrence of large numbers of epithelioid histiocytes, eosinophils, and plasma cells. The absence of polyclonal staining may indicate that the process is not reactive. Excisional biopsy is strongly recommended in problematic cases.[41] It may be difficult to differentiate between peripheral T-cell lymphomas and Hodgkin's disease.

Occasionally, atypical mononuclear and binucleated cells resembling Reed-Sternberg cells have been observed in T cell lymphomas. The presence of numerous atypical mononucleated and binucleated cells that stain positively for Leu-M1 and negatively for LCA, although not specific, favors Hodgkin's disease.[3]

Hodgkin's Disease

Hodgkin's disease is the most common type of lymphoma that occurs in young adults. Histologically, Hodgkin's disease is subclassified as lymphocytic predominant, nodular sclerosing, mixed cellularity, and lymphocytic depleted. Evidence has emerged to warrant recognition of lymphocytic-predominant Hodgkin's disease as a distinct entity. Although it consists of neoplastic cells in a background of benign inflammatory cells, similar to other subtypes, it differs morphologically, immunophenotypically, and clinically from classic Hodgkin's disease. To distinguish this tumor from the diffuse lym-

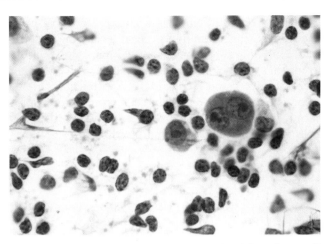

FIG. 4-40. Hodgkin's disease. A classic Reed-Sternberg cell is present. (Papanicolaou stain, ×800)

phocyte predominance in the Rye classification, the term *paragranuloma* has been proposed.[40]

Cytopathology

The cytologic diagnosis of Hodgkin's disease is based on the demonstration of classic Reed-Sternberg cells in the appropriate reactive background. Reed-Sternberg cells are large binucleated or multinucleated cells that contain nuclei with reticulated chromatin and prominent macronucleoli (Figs. 4-39 and 4-40). Although the cytoplasm is abundant, the nucleus often appears as if it is surrounded by an empty space because the cytoplasm is pale and fragile. Cases that do not have classic Reed-Sternberg cells or that demonstrate only Hodgkin's cells (large mononucleated cells with reticulated chromatin and one to two prominent nucleoli) require histologic examination for a definitive diagnosis.

Although some investigators[53,54] have subtyped Hodgkin's disease according to the relative proportions of neoplastic cells (Hodgkin's and Reed-Sternberg cells) and reactive cellular components on cytologic preparations, histologic examination is necessary to distinguish subtypes with confidence. Lymphocytic-predominant (paragranuloma) Hodgkin's disease is characterized by a predominance of small lymphocytes with large atypical lobulated mononucleated or "popcorn" cells. Reed-Sternberg cells, eosinophils, and plasma cells are rare to absent. Epithelioid histiocytes are often present in small clusters. Aspirates of nodular sclerosing Hodgkin's disease contain classic Reed-Sternberg cells, lacunar cells, eosinophils, lymphocytes, and histiocytes. Lacunar cells are large cells with abundant clear or pale cytoplasm containing indented or overlapping segmented nuclei; these cells are not specific for Hodgkin's disease. The syncytial variant of nodular sclerosing Hodgkin's disease shows numerous atypical mononuclear cells. Mixed cellularity

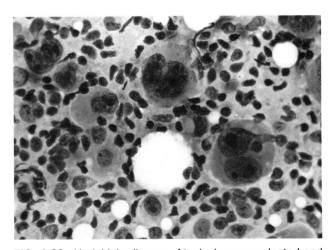

FIG. 4-39. Hodgkin's disease. Atypical mononucleated and binucleated cells are present in a background of lymphocytes. (Diff-Quik stain, ×500)

Hodgkin's disease demonstrates Reed-Sternberg cells, Hodgkin's cells, eosinophils, plasma cells, histiocytes, and lymphocytes. Aspirates of lymphocytic-depleted Hodgkin's disease may be scantly cellular and consist of Reed-Sternberg and Hodgkin's cells with a sparse lymphoid component or spindle cells representing fibroblastic proliferation. The Reed-Sternberg and Hodgkin's cells may show marked pleomorphism.

Ancillary Studies

Most Reed-Sternberg cells and their variants stain positively for Leu-M1 and Ki-1, except for those in lymphocytic-predominant Hodgkin's disease (paragranuloma), and negatively for CD20 and CD45. The many of lymphocytes in Hodgkin's disease are nonneoplastic and have a T-cell origin.

Cytokinetic studies usually show a diploid population with a low proliferation index. About 10% of cases show a tetraploid or hypertetraploid cell population that corresponds to an increased number of Reed-Sternberg cells.

Differential Diagnosis

T-cell lymphoma, reactive hyperplasia, poorly differentiated carcinoma, and sarcoma are diagnostic considerations. Large binucleated cells resembling Reed-Sternberg cells have been described in non-Hodgkin's large cell lymphoma and in nonneoplastic reactive conditions. Pleomorphic high-grade T-cell lymphomas may contain large atypical mononuclear cells resembling Reed-Sternberg cell variants in a background of small T cells and may be difficult to differentiate from Hodgkin's disease. The background lymphocytes in Hodgkin's disease are rounder and less irregular than those in T-cell lymphoma; however, this may be a subtle distinguishing feature. Both pleomorphic T-cell lymphoma and Hodgkin's disease may show a predominance of helper T cells. Ki-1 antibody is not a reliable discriminator because it may stain both Hodgkin's cells and malignant T cells. Aberrant staining of T cells is demonstrated by the loss of the pan–T-cell antigen and may be indicative of a neoplastic T cell process. In some cases gene rearrangement studies may be helpful in distinguishing between T-cell lymphoma or anaplastic large cell lymphoma and Hodgkin's disease by demonstrating rearrangement of the T-cell receptor genes in the former and a germline pattern in Hodgkin's disease.

Atypical immunoblasts in reactive processes such as infectious mononucleosis, postvaccinal lymphadenitis, and Dilantin hypersensitivity lymphadenopathy may resemble Reed-Sternberg cells and atypical mononuclear cells; however, they usually have coarser chromatin and smaller nucleoli than those in cells in Hodgkin's dis-

ease.[27,28] Both reactive and neoplastic conditions demonstrate polyclonality and have a similar ploidy pattern. Clusters of epithelioid histiocytes may also occur in both processes.

Lymphocytic-depleted or the syncytial variant of nodular sclerosing Hodgkin's disease may be mistaken for poorly differentiated carcinoma or anaplastic large cell lymphoma. Positive immunostaining for keratin would be helpful in separating the former. The distinction between lymphocytic-depleted/syncytial variant of Hodgkin's disease and anaplastic large cell lymphoma may be impossible by cytologic evaluation.

METASTATIC TUMORS IN LYMPH NODES

Lymph nodes clinically suspected of metastatic disease are one of the most common indications for FNA. In patients with enlarging lymph nodes and previous documented malignancy, FNA can obviate further surgery performed merely to confirm metastasis. FNA may be performed to stage malignancies, particularly in patients who are high risk for surgery. In patients without a previous diagnosis, FNA can not only confirm the presence of metastatic disease but also give clues to the nature of the tumor and suggest possible primary sites of origin. When evaluating lymph node metastases in cases with an unknown primary tumor, it is helpful to pose the question, "Which neoplasms have a predilection to metastasize to this particular site in a patient of this age and sex?" (Table 4-3). Even though the patient has a documented history of a primary neoplasm, the physician should consider the possibility of a new primary tumor and determine whether the cytomorphology of the me-

TABLE 4-3. *Sources of neoplasms that frequently metastasize to lymph nodes*

CERVICAL	MEDIASTINAL
Oral cavity	Lung
Naropharynx	
Thyroid	AXILLARY
Larynx	Breast
Skin of face	Skin (melanoma)
SUPRACLAVICULAR/SCALENE	ABDOMINAL
Head and neck (squamous carcinoma)	Gastrointestinal tract
Lung	Kidney
Ovary	Gonads
Skin (melanoma)	Uterine body
Renal	
Prostate	PELVIC
	Cervix
INGUINAL	Uterine body
Skin (melanoma)	Prostate
Cervix	
Vulva or perineum	
Anal canal or rectum	

tastasis corresponds with the known primary neoplasm. It is always helpful to compare the previous surgical or cytologic specimen with the current one.

Squamous Carcinoma

Aspirates of metastatic squamous carcinoma show cohesive epithelial groups with variable numbers of keratinizing cells, depending on the degree of differentiation. Keratinizing tumors have abundant, sharply demarcated, dense orangeophilic cytoplasm on Papanicolaou stained smears (Fig. 4-41). On air-dried smears stained with Diff-Quik, the cytoplasm is royal blue. Structures suggesting epithelial "pearls" or cells arranged in a cell-in-cell (bird's eye) pattern may be seen. Tumor cells may be round, oval, polygonal, or spindle- or tadpole-shaped. Anucleated squames may also occur. Nuclei are round to oval and hyperchromatic with coarsely granular chromatin. Nucleoli may occasionally be observed.

In well-differentiated squamous carcinoma, the tumor cells may closely resemble normal squamous cells. In such cases, the differential diagnosis includes branchial cleft cyst and keratinous cyst. Branchial cleft cysts are located in the lateral aspect of the neck and may suddenly become palpable in adult life. Aspirates show mature squamous cells, anucleated squames, and lymphocytes in a background of proteinaceous material. Occasionally, small immature squamous cells with atypia may be present mimicking carcinoma. In the absence of carcinoma in the head and neck region or thorax, aspirates should be interpreted cautiously and recommend surgical excision. Clinical history can be helpful in differentiating keratinous cysts, which are usually present for a long time without significant change. Aspirates of keratinous cysts show mature squamous cells and anucleated squames.

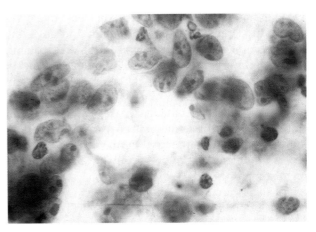

FIG. 4-42. Nasopharyngeal carcinoma. Posterior cervical aspirate shows cohesive groups of poorly differentiated tumor cells. (Papanicolaou stain, ×1000)

Nasopharyngeal Carcinoma

Nasopharyngeal carcinomas are subtyped as keratinizing squamous cell carcinoma (type 1), nonkeratinizing carcinoma (type 2), and undifferentiated carcinoma (lymphoepithelioma). Not infrequently, the primary tumor is clinically occult and the initial presentation is an enlarged posterior cervical lymph node. It has a bimodal age distribution with one peak occurring in adolescents and young adults and another peak in older adults. Epstein-Barr virus has been associated with both nonkeratinizing and undifferentiated nasopharyngeal carcinoma.[55]

Aspirates show a poorly differentiated tumor cells arranged in cohesive groups (Fig. 4-42) or singly (Fig. 4-43). In the dispersed single cell (Schminke) variant of lymphoepithelioma, the cells may resemble the mononuclear variants of Hodgkin's disease. Tumor cells are

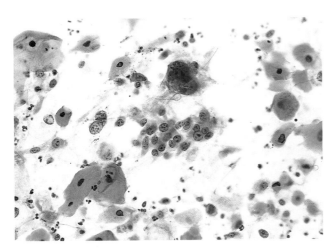

FIG. 4-41. Metastatic squamous carcinoma. Lymph node aspirate from a patient with a lung mass shows atypical keratinizing and nonkeratinizing cells. (Papanicolaou stain, ×320)

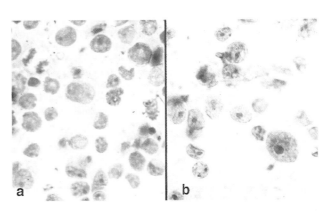

FIG. 4-43. Nasopharyngeal carcinoma. Air-dried (**A**) and alcohol-fixed (**B**) smears show a dispersed population of tumor cells that may be mistaken for a high-grade lymphoma or Hodgkin's disease. (**A**, Diff-Quik stain, ×1000; **B**, Papanicolaou stain, ×1000)

large and moderately pleomorphic. Nuclei are oval with finely to moderately granular chromatin and have one to two prominent central nucleoli. Mitoses are frequent. The cytoplasmic borders are often ill defined, resulting in a syncytial appearance. Small cleaved lymphocytes are often admixed with the tumor cells.[56]

The tumor cells in nasopharyngeal carcinomas are keratin positive. Ultrastructural analysis demonstrates tonofilaments and well-formed desmosomes. The presence of tonofilaments indicating squamous differentiation distinguishes this tumor from other carcinomas such as adenocarcinoma and embryonal carcinoma. Although nasopharyngeal carcinoma has also been called lymphoepithelioma, this is somewhat of a misnomer because the lymphocytes associated with the tumor are benign. It is a reminder, however, that nasopharyngeal carcinoma is often difficult to distinguish from lymphoma. The key is to think of nasopharyngeal carcinoma in the differential diagnosis.

Adenocarcinoma

Aspirates of adenocarcinoma usually show tumor cells arranged in cohesive groups (Fig. 4-44) and singly, regardless of the site of origin. Cell groups may consist of ball-like clusters, papillary fragments, loose clusters, or acini with central lumen. Tumor cells may be round, cuboidal, or columnar in shape. Nuclei often have a vesicular chromatin and prominent nucleoli. The cytoplasm may vary in appearance from homogenous to markedly vacuolated. The vacuoles may be small and numerous or large, resulting in margination and indentation of the nucleus.

Some cases of metastatic adenocarcinoma contain certain cytologic features that may give clues to the site of

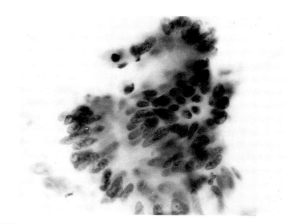

FIG. 4-45. Metastatic colon carcinoma. Lymph node aspirate shows atypical columnar cells with elongated palisading nuclei. (Papanicolaou stain, ×500) Although not pictured, necrosis is usually present in the background.

the primary tumor. The presence of columnar cells with elongated palisading nuclei in a necrotic background suggest a colonic primary tumor (Fig. 4-45). Signet-ring cells with intracytoplasmic mucin are commonly associated with a gastric primary tumor, but may be seen in other primary tumors (Fig. 4-46). Characteristically, intracytoplasmic mucin has a targetoid appearance. The Mayer mucicarmine stain is helpful in demonstrating intracytoplasmic mucin and can be performed on destained Papanicolaou-stained smears. In general, the presence of intracytoplasmic mucin excludes hepatocellular, renal, adrenal, and thyroid carcinoma. A renal primary tumor may be suggested if the cells are large with abundant granular or finely vacuolated cytoplasm and have round nuclei with prominent nucleoli (Fig. 4-47). Renal cell carcinoma can metastasize many years after the primary tumor is diagnosed. Glandular cells ar-

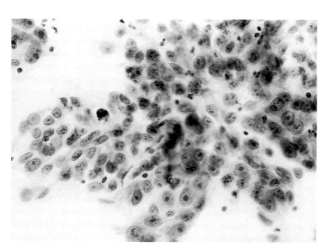

FIG. 4-44. Metastatic adenocarcinoma. Lymph node aspirate from a patient with lung carcinoma shows a cohesive group of cells with oval nuclei, vesicular chromatin, and prominent nucleoli. (Papanicolaou stain, ×320)

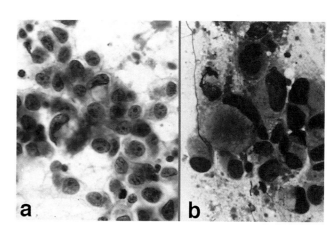

FIG. 4-46. Metastatic signet-ring carcinoma. Alcohol-fixed (A) and air-dried (B) smears show tumor cells with vacuoles causing indentation and margination of the nucleus. (A, Papanicolaou stain, ×320; B, Diff-Quik stain, ×500)

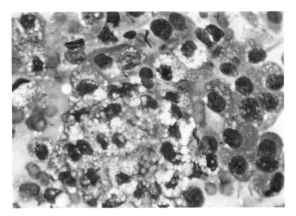

FIG. 4-47. Metastatic renal cell carcinoma. Tumors have abundant, finely vacuolated cytoplasm and round nuclei. (Diff-Quik stain, ×400)

ranged in a cribriform pattern with round nuclei and prominent nucleoli suggest a prostatic primary tumor. Positive immunostaining for prostate-specific antigen or prostatic acid phosphatase or both is helpful in supporting this diagnosis. Butler and colleagues[57] described supraclavicular metastases as the initial presentation of prostate carcinoma. Papillary fragments containing enlarged nuclei with fine powdery chromatin, micro- or macronucleoli, nuclear grooves, and intranuclear cytoplasmic inclusions are in keeping with a thyroid primary tumor, particularly if aspirated from a cervical lymph node. Psammoma bodies may be associated with papillary carcinomas and have been described in metastases primarily from thyroid, ovary, lung, and endometrial tumors.

Undifferentiated Small Cell Carcinoma

Aspirates of undifferentiated small cell carcinoma show small cells arranged in loose clusters and singly.

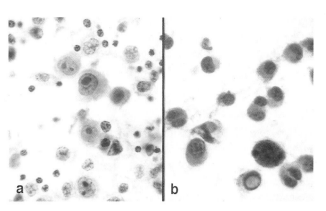

FIG. 4-49. Metastatic melanoma. (A) Aspirate consists of a dispersed population of cells with moderately abundant cytoplasm, round to oval nuclei, and prominent nucleoli. (Papanicolaou stain, ×500) (B) Tumor cells contain melanin pigment and intranuclear cytoplasmic inclusions. (Papanicolaou stain, ×500)

Tumors cells are one and one half to two times larger than the size of lymphocytes. The cytoplasm is scant. Nuclei may vary from round to irregular. The nuclear chromatin is finely granular but hyperchromatic and at times pyknotic (Fig. 4-48). Nucleoli are small and inconspicuous. The presence of aggregates of cells showing cell molding and individual cell necrosis (apoptosis) are characteristic of small cell carcinoma and helpful in distinguishing it from lymphoma.

Melanoma

Cytomorphologically, melanoma can show a variety of features and is known as the "great mimicker." Aspirates are usually cellular and consist primarily of a dispersed population of cells with occasional cell clustering. Tumor cells are usually round to polygonal but can be spindle shaped (Figs. 4-49 and 4-50). The round to po-

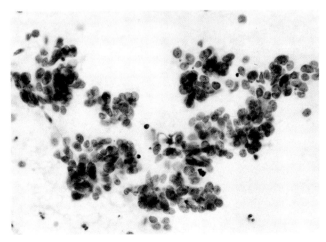

FIG. 4-48. Metastatic undifferentiated small cell carcinoma. Aspirate from a cervical lymph node shows small tumor cells with scant cytoplasm, nuclear molding, and a fine chromatin pattern. (Papanicolaou stain, ×400)

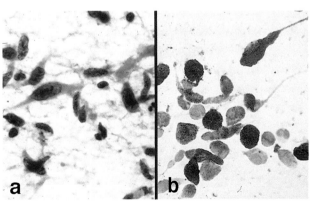

FIG. 4-50. Metastatic melanoma. (A) A predominantly spindled cell population may be seen in melanoma. (Papanicolaou stain, ×500) (B) Positive immunostaining for HMB-45 is helpful in confirming the diagnosis. (Immunoperoxidase stain, ×500)

lygonal tumor cells have abundant cytoplasm with well-defined cell borders. Mirror-image binucleated and multinucleated cells are often present. Most cells have a plasmacytoid appearance with eccentrically located nuclei; this feature is more pronounced on Diff-Quik preparations. Nuclei are round to pleomorphic, have finely granular chromatin, and either have one prominent nucleolus or two to three smaller nucleoli. Intranuclear cytoplasmic inclusions are commonly seen.

The presence of finely granular pigment in the cytoplasm of malignant cells is helpful in cases suspected of metastatic melanoma; however, between 30% to 60% of aspirates from melanomas may be amelanotic.[58] In these cases, melanin pigment should be differentiated from hemosiderin, which is a coarser pigment.

A number of morphologic variants of melanoma have been described, including a signet-ring configuration, pseudopapillary, small cell, and myxoid patterns.[59] It is often helpful to compare the cytomorphologic features of the metastasis with those of the primary tumor. In the absence of histologically confirmed melanoma, a definitive cytologic diagnosis of metastatic melanoma should be confirmed by immunocytochemical studies that show positive staining for HMB-45 or ultrastructural analysis that demonstrates premelanosomes.

Germ Cell Tumors

Aspirates of seminoma show a predominantly dispersed population of large monomorphous cells admixed with small mature lymphocytes (Fig. 4-51). Tumor cells are large with scant to moderate cytoplasm. Occasionally, cells contain multiple small cytoplasmic vacuoles readily identified on Diff-Quik smears. Nuclei are round to slightly irregular, have finely granular chro-

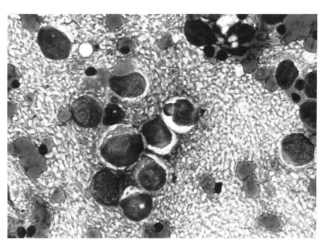

FIG. 4-52. Metastatic seminoma. The presence of a tigroid background is a helpful diagnostic feature. (Diff-Quik stain, ×400)

matin, and have one prominent central nucleolus. Variable numbers of lymphocytes, plasma cells, and epithelioid histiocytes are present in the background. The tigroid background (Fig. 4-52) seen on Diff-Quik preparations is a helpful diagnostic feature; however, it is only seen in 38% of cases.[60] The differential diagnosis in cases of an unknown primary tumor include large cell lymphoma, nonseminomatous tumors, metastatic melanoma, and metastatic adenocarcinoma. Immunocytochemical studies may be helpful in distinguishing these entities. Seminoma usually shows positive staining for placental alkaline phosphatase (PLAP) and negative staining for LCA, Ki-1, HMB-45, and keratin.[61]

Both embryonal and endodermal sinus tumors show a papillary or glandlike arrangement of cells. Nuclei are large and pleomorphic with one to three nucleoli (Fig. 4-53). An endodermal sinus tumor also has markedly

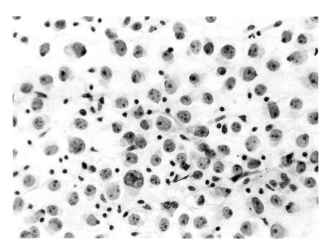

FIG. 4-51. Metastatic seminoma. Smear shows a dispersed population of tumor cells with round nuclei and central prominent nucleoli admixed with small lymphocytes. (Papanicolaou stain, ×300)

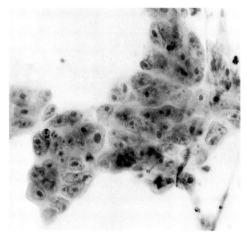

FIG. 4-53. Metastatic embryonal carcinoma. Supraclavicular lymph node aspirate in a young man shows cohesive large cells with pleomorphic nuclei and prominent nucleoli. (Papanicolaou stain, ×300)

vacuolated cytoplasm that may contain homogeneous hyalin inclusions.[62,63] An embryonal carcinoma shows positive immunostaining for low molecular-weight keratin, PLAP, and Ki-l. An endodermal sinus tumor demonstrates positivity for α-fetoprotein.

Although adequate sampling of germ cell tumors is helpful in detecting more than one component, a mixed germ cell tumor cannot be totally excluded on cytologic evaluation alone. The cytologic findings must be correlated with the clinical findings, including serum α-fetoprotein and human choriogonadotropin.

Sarcoma

In general, sarcomas rarely metastasize to lymph nodes; however, the sarcomas that do include rhabdomyosarcoma, Kaposi's sarcoma, clear cell sarcoma (malignant melanoma of soft parts), epithelioid sarcoma, and angiosarcoma. Embryonal rhabdomyosarcoma is important because it commonly metastasizes to lymph nodes and this may be the first sign of disease; thus it must be differentiated from other small round cell tumors of childhood including lymphoma. Aspirates show a dispersed cell population with variable cytomorphology not only from case to case but within the same tumor. Tumor cells often are small with thin rims of cytoplasm; however, larger cells with abundant cytoplasm and eccentrically located nuclei may also be present. Spindle or ribbon-shaped cells are sometimes seen.[64] Most rhabdomyosarcomas are positive for desmin. Ultrastructural analysis shows thick and thin filaments with attempts at Z-band formation.

Kaposi's sarcoma develops in about one third of patients who have acquired immunodeficiency syndrome. Aspirates often show fragments of spindle cells with ill-defined cytoplasmic borders and nuclear overlap (Fig. 4-54); loosely cohesive and individual spindle-shaped cells are also present.[65] Aspirates of clear cell sarcoma show round to polygonal tumor cells with moderately abundant cytoplasm and round nuclei with prominent nucleoli. Because the cytologic as well as the immunocytochemical and ultrastructural features are indistinguishable from those of metastatic melanoma, clinical correlation is necessary.[66] Aspirates of epithelioid sarcoma can show a spectrum of cytologic features ranging from histiocytic cells mimicking a granulomatous process to tadpole-shaped cells mimicking squamous carcinoma.[67] Cutaneous angiosarcoma occurring in the head and neck area commonly metastasizes to the cervical lymph nodes.[68] Aspirates of angiosarcoma show spindle to polygonal cells with pleomorphism. Tumor cells may form papillary tufts or microacinar structures.[69] Positive immunostaining for vimentin, factor VIII-related antigen, and *Ulex europaeus* agglutinin-1 may be helpful in supporting this diagnosis.

REFERENCES

1. Cohen MB, Miller TR, Bottles K. Classics in cytology: note on fine needle aspiration of the lymphatic glands in sleeping sickness (Letter) Acta Cytol 1986; 30:451.
2. Guthrie CG. Gland puncture as a diagnostic measure. Bull Johns Hopkins Hosp 1921; 32:266.
3. Katz RL. Cytologic diagnosis of leukemia and lymphoma: values and limitations. Clin Lab Med 1991; 11:469.
4. Shaha A, Webber C, Marti J. Fine-needle aspiration in the diagnosis of lymphadenopathy. Am J Surg 1986; 152:420.
5. Gupta AK, Nayar M, Chandra M. Reliability and limitations of fine needle aspiration cytology of lymphadenopathies. Acta Cytol 1991; 35:777.
6. Pilotti S, Di Palma S, Alasio L, et al. Diagnostic assessment of enlarged superficial lymph nodes by fine needle aspiration. Acta Cytol 1993; 37:853.
7. Steel BL, Schwartz MR, Ramzy I. Fine needle aspiration biopsy in the diagnosis of lymphadenopathy in 1,103 patients: role, limitations and analysis of diagnostic pitfalls. Acta Cytol 1995; 39:76.
8. Sneige N. Diagnosis of lymphoma and reactive lymphoid hyperplasia by immunocytochemical analysis of fine-needle aspiration biopsy. Diagn Cytopathol 1990; 6:39.
9. Sneige N, Dekmezian RH, Katz RL, et al. Morphologic and immunocytochemical evaluation of 220 fine needle aspirates of malignant lymphoma and lymphoid hyperplasia. Acta Cytol 1990; 34: 311.
10. Robins DB, Katz RL, Swan F, et al. Immunophenotyping of lymphoma by fine-needle aspiration: a comparative study of cytospin preparations and flow cytometry. Am J Clin Pathol 1994; 10:569.
11. Tsang WY, Chan JK. Spectrum of morphologic changes in lymph nodes attributable to fine needle aspiration. Hum Pathol 1992; 23: 562.
12. Dekmezian RH, Sneige N, Katz RL. The effect of fine needle aspiration on lymph node morphology in lymphoproliferative disorders. Acta Cytol 1989; 33:732.
13. Behm FG, O'Dowd GJ, Frable WJ. Fine-needle aspiration effects on benign lymph node histology. Am J Clin Pathol 1984; 82:195.
14. Cleary KR, Osborne BM, Butler JJ. Lymph node infarction foreshadowing malignant lymphoma. Am Surg Pathol 1982; 6:435.
15. Katz RL, Caraway NP. FNA lymphoproliferative diseases: myths and legends. Diagn Cytopathol 1995; 12:99.
16. Shabb N, Katz RL, Ordonez NG, et al. Fine-needle aspiration evaluation of lymphoproliferative lesions in human immunodeficiency virus-positive patients. Cancer 1991; 67:1008.
17. Ioachim HL. Lymph node pathology. Philadelphia: JB Lippincott, 1994:137.
18. Rajwanshi A, Bhambhani S, Das DK. Fine-needle aspiration cytology diagnosis of tuberculosis. Diagn Cytopathol 1987; 3:13.

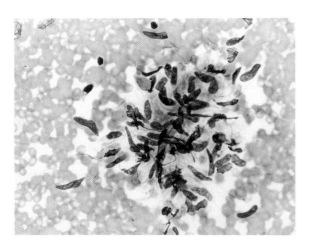

FIG. 4-54. Kaposi's sarcoma. Lymph node aspirate from a patient infected with HIV shows a fragment composed of spindled cells with hyperchromatic nuclei. (Diff-Quik stain, ×500)

19. Pandit AA, Khilnani PH, Prayag AS. Tuberculous lymphadenitis: extended cytomorphologic features. Diagn Cytopathol 1995;12:23.

20. Ang GAT, Janda WM, Novak RM, et al. Negative images of mycobacteria in aspiration biopsy smears from the lymph node of a patient with acquired immunodeficiency syndrome (AIDS): report of a case and review of the literature. Diagn Cytopathol 1993;9:325.

21. Stanley MW, Horwitz CA, Burton LG, et al. Negative images of bacilli and mycobacterial infection: a study of fine-needle aspiration smears from lymph nodes in patients with AIDS. Diagn Cytopathol 1990;6:118.

22. Gupta SK, Kumar B, Kaur S. Aspiration cytology in lymph nodes in leprosy. Int J Lepr Other Mycobact Dis 1981;49:9.

23. Myerowitz RL. Local and disseminated cryptococcoses. In: Myerowitz RL, ed. The pathology of opportunistic infections. New York, Raven Press, 1983:145.

24. Baker RD. The primary pulmonary lymph node complex of cryptococcoses. Am J Clin Pathol 1976;65:83.

25. Alfonso F, Gallo L, Winkler B, et al. Fine needle aspiration cytology of peripheral lymph node cryptococcoses: a report of three cases. Acta Cytol 1994;38:459.

26. Strigle SM, Rarick MU, Cosgrove MM, et al. A review of the fine-needle aspiration cytology findings in human immunodeficiency virus infection. Diagn Cytopathol 1992;8:41.

27. Stanley MW, Steeper TA, Horwitz CA, et al. Fine-needle aspiration of lymph nodes in patients with acute infectious mononucleosis. Diagn Cytopathol 1990;6:323.

28. Kardos TF, Kornstein MJ, Frable WJ. Cytology and immunocytology of infectious mononucleosis in fine needle aspirates of lymph nodes. Acta Cytol 1988;32:722.

29. Ewing EP, Chandler FW, Spira TJ, et al. Primary lymph node pathology in AIDS and AIDS-related lymphadenopathy. Arch Pathol Lab Med 1985;109:977.

30. Pallesen G, Gerstoft J, Mathiesen L. Stages in LAV/HTLV-III lymphadenitis: histological and immunologic classification. Scand J Immunol 1987;25:83.

31. Oertel J, Oertel B, Lobeck H, et al. Immunocytochemical analysis of lymph node aspirates in patients with human immunodeficiency virus infection. J Clin Pathol 1990;43:844.

32. Martin-Bates E, Tanner A, Suvarna SK, et al. Use of fine needle aspiration cytology for investigating lymphadenopathy in HIV positive patients. J Clin Pathol 1993;46:564.

33. Argyle JC, Schumann GB, Kjeldsberg CR, et al. Identification of a toxoplasma cyst by fine needle aspiration. Am J Clin Pathol 1983;80:256.

34. Frable MA, Frable WJ. Fine-needle aspiration biopsy: efficacy in the diagnosis of head and neck sarcoidosis. Laryngoscope 1984;94:1281.

35. Morales CF, Patefield AJ, Strollo PJ, et al. Flexible transbronchial needle aspiration in the diagnosis of sarcoidosis. Chest 1994;106:709.

36. Perez-Guillermo M, Sola Perez J, Espinosa Parra FJ. Asteroid bodies and calcium oxalate crystals: two infrequent findings in fine-needle aspirates of parotid sarcoidosis. Diagn Cytopathol 1992;8:248.

37. Stansfeld AG, Diebold J, Kapanci Y, et al. Updated Kiel classification for lymphomas. Lancet 1988;1:292.

38. Lennert K, Feller AC. Histopathology of non-Hodgkin's lymphomas, ed 2. New York, Springer-Verlag, 1992.

39. Non-Hodgkin's lymphoma pathologic classification project. National Cancer Institute sponsored study of classifications of non-Hodgkin's lymphomas: summary and description of a Working Formulation for clinical usage. Cancer 1982;49:2112.

40. Harris NL, Jaffe ES, Stein H, et al. A revised European-American classification of lymphoid neoplasms: a proposal from the international lymphoma study group. Blood 1994;84:1361.

41. Katz RL, Gritsman A, Cabanillas F, et al. Fine-needle aspiration cytology of peripheral T-cell lymphoma. Am J Clin Pathol 1989;91:120.

42. Katz RL, Wojcik EM, Johnston DA. Image analysis in non-Hodgkin's lymphomas emphasizing applications in tissue procured by fine needle aspiration. In: Wied GL, Bartels PH, Rosenthal DL, Schenck U, eds. The compendium on the computerized cytology and histology laboratory. Chicago, Tutorials of Cytology, 1994:241.

43. Wojcik EM, Katz RL, Fanning TV, et al. Diagnosis of mantle cell lymphoma on tissue acquired by FNA in conjunction with immunocytochemistry and cytokinetic studies: possibilities and limitations. Acta Cytol 1995;39:909.

44. Erler BS, Katz RK. Accurate diagnosis of low cytologic grade B cell lymphomas in fine needle aspirates using cytomorphologic, immunophenotypic, and proliferation marker studies. Mod Pathol 1995;8:39A.

45. Collins RD, Casey TT, Glick AD, et al. B-cell neoplasms. In: Sternberg SS, ed. Diagnostic surgical pathology, vol 1. New York, Raven Press, 1989:541.

46. Dorform DM, Pinkus GS. Distinction between small lymphoctyic and mantle cell lymphoma by immunoreactivity for CD23. Mod Pathol 1994;7:326.

47. Lardelli P, Bookman MA, Sundeen J, et al. Lymphocytic lymphoma of intermediate differentiation: morphologic and immunophenotypic spectrum and clinical correlations. Am J Surg Pathol 1990;14:752.

48. Mann RB, Berard CW. Criteria for the cytologic subclassification of follicular lymphomas: a proposed alternative method. Hematol Oncol 1983;1:187.

49. Ngan B, Chen-Levy Z, Weiss LM, et al. Expression in non-Hodgkin's lymphoma of the bcl-2 protein associated with the t(14;18) chromosomal translocation. N Engl J Med 1988;318:1638.

50. Pezzella F, Tse AGD, Cordell JL, et al. Expression of the bcl-2 oncogene protein is not specific for the 14;18 chromosomal translocation. Am J Pathol 1990;137:225.

51. Jacobs JC, Katz RL, Shabb N, et al. Fine needle aspiration of lymphoblastic lymphoma. Acta Cytol 1992;36:887.

52. Weis JW, Winter MW, Phyliky RL, et al. Peripheral T-cell lymphomas: histologic, immunohistologic, and clinical characterization. Mayo Clin Proc 1986;61:411.

53. Das DK, Gupta SK, Datta BN, et al. Fine needle aspiration cytodiagnosis of Hodgkin's disease and its subtypes. I. Scope and limitations. Acta Cytol 1990;34:329.

54. Das DK, Gupta SK. Fine needle aspiration cytodiagnosis of Hodgkin's disease and its subtypes. II. Subtyping by differential cell counts. Acta Cytol 1990;34:337.

55. Mills SE, Fechner RE. The nose, paranasal sinuses, and nasopharynx. In: Sternberg SS, ed. Diagnostic surgical pathology, vol 1. New York, Raven Press, 1989:666.

56. Grenco RT, Shabb NS. Metastatic nasopharyngeal carcinoma: cytologic features of 18 cases. Diagn Cytopathol 1991;7:562.

57. Butler JJ, Howe CD, Johnson DE. Enlargement of the supraclavicular lymph nodes as the initial sign of prostatic carcinoma. Cancer 1971;27:1055.

58. Layfield LJ, Ostrzega N. Fine needle aspirate smear morphology in metastatic melanoma. Acta Cytol 1989;33:606.

59. Nakhleh RE, Wick MR, Rocamora A, et al. Morphologic diversity in malignant melanomas. Am J Clin Pathol 1990;93:731.

60. Caraway NP, Fanning CV, Amato RJ, et al. Fine-needle aspiration cytology of seminoma: a review of 16 cases. Diagn Cytopathol 1995;12:327.

61. Young RH, Scully RE. Testicular tumors. Chicago, ASCP Press, 1990:12.

62. Balslev E, Francis D, Jacobsen GK. Testicular germ cell tumors: classification based on fine needle aspiration biopsy. Acta Cytol 1990;34:690.

63. Akhtar M, Ali MA, Sackey K, et al. Fine-needle aspiration biopsy diagnosis of endodermal sinus tumor. Diagn Cytopathol 1990;6:184.

64. Seidal T, Walaas L, Kindblom L-G, et al. Cytology of embryonal rhabdomyosarcoma. Diagn Cytopathol 1988;4:292.

65. Hales M, Bottles K, Miller T, et al. Diagnosis of Kaposi's sarcoma by fine-needle aspiration biopsy. Am J Clin Pathol 1987;88:20.

66. Caraway NP, Fanning CV, Wojcik EM, et al. Cytology of malignant melanoma of soft parts. Diagn Cytopathol 1993;9:632.

67. Goswitz JJ, Kappel T, Klingaman K. Fine-needle aspiration of epithelioid sarcoma. Diagn Cytopathol 1993;9:677.

68. Enzinger FM, Weis SW. Soft tissue tumors. St Louis, Mosby, 1988:545.

69. Silverman JF, Lannin DL, Larkin EW, et al. Fine-needle aspiration cytology of postradiation sarcoma, including angiosarcoma, with immunocytochemical confirmation. Diagn Cytopathol 1989;5:281.

Fine Needle Aspiration of Subcutaneous Organs and Masses,
edited by Yener S. Erozan and Thomas A. Bonfiglio.
Lippincott–Raven Publishers, Philadelphia, © 1996.

CHAPTER 5

Fine Needle Aspiration of the Thyroid Gland

John R. Goellner

Aspiration cytologic study of the thyroid has become an important diagnostic procedure in the management of thyroid abnormalities. Cytologic study can detect the presence of malignancy and can usually predict the cell type. In some cases, this information obviates a surgical procedure. In other cases, this knowledge guides the preoperative evaluation and the choice of surgical procedure. If the lesion or abnormality is not malignant, cytologic study often can categorize the benign state that is present—for example, Hashimoto's thyroiditis or subacute thyroiditis.

Interpretation of thyroid cytologic features, as with any other organ site, is predicated on an understanding of the normal anatomy and histology and the pathologic states of the thyroid gland.

THYROID ANATOMY: GROSS AND MICROSCOPIC

The thyroid is located in the anterior region of the neck, in front and on both sides of the trachea. It is closely associated with the trachea and with the neurovascular bundles of the lateral neck and also is invested with lymph nodes. Cells aspirated from a thyroid mass actually may be from structures adjacent to the thyroid gland. Histologically, the normal thyroid gland is composed of spherical units of epithelial cells surrounding a

gelatinous protein-hormone material referred to as *colloid*. The consistency of the colloid may vary, depending on the physiologic state of the gland, from a thin watery material to much more solid globules.

The cells lining the thyroid follicles are epithelial cells that elaborate the thyroglobulin. Normally, they are low cuboidal cells and appear to be inactive cytologically with small, regular nuclei showing even, finely granular chromatin and inconspicuous nucleoli; their cytoplasm is scanty. C cells are scattered among the follicle lining cells, and they produce thyrocalcitonin. C cells lie within the basement membrane of the follicles but generally do not reach the lumen of the follicle, like the Kulchitsky cell of the gastrointestinal tract, to which C cells are related within the neuroendocrine group.

The stromal framework for the follicular units is composed of blood vessels and small amounts of fibrous tissue, analogous in many ways to the interstitial tissue of pulmonary parenchyma. In disease states, the stromal mesenchymal tissues may increase in amount as a result of fibrosis, edema, or inflammation.

OUTLINE OF THYROID PATHOLOGY

A useful classification divides thyroid pathology as related to aspiration cytology into three main groups: goiter, thyroiditis, and neoplasm.

The term *goiter* refers to an enlargement of the thyroid gland, and the common division is into two types: toxic and nontoxic. In toxic goiter, the gland is diffusely en-

J. R. Goellner: Division of Anatomic Pathology, Mayo Clinic and Mayo Foundation, Rochester, MN 55905.

larged and is overactive, producing a hypermetabolic state referred to as *hyperthyroidism* or *Graves' disease.* Nontoxic goiters are commonly referred to as *multinodular goiters*; the thyroid is enlarged either symmetrically or asymmetrically and is variably nodular on physical examination, but the patient is euthyroid metabolically.

Thyroiditis is divided into three forms: lymphocytic or Hashimoto's thyroiditis, subacute or de Quervain's thyroiditis, and fibrous or Riedel's thyroiditis. Hashimoto's thyroiditis is common in the United States and may present clinically in various forms. Some patients have the disease for some years and are in a hypothyroid state because of loss of functional thyroid parenchyma when they are first seen for diagnosis. Others may present with an enlarged thyroid gland (goiter). Sometimes there is an associated hyperthyroid state due to uncontrolled release of hormone secondary to disruption of the gland.

De Quervain's thyroiditis is also referred to as *subacute thyroiditis* or *granulomatous thyroiditis.* Patients with this disease generally present with a tender, painful nodule in the thyroid, which may have developed after a viral illness. The nodule persists for weeks and then may resolve spontaneously.

Riedel's thyroiditis is a very rare disease in which the thyroid gland is replaced by inflammation and dense fibrosis that extend into the surrounding tissues. This disease is considered to be related to idiopathic retroperitoneal fibrosis, sclerosing mediastinitis, and other similar conditions.

Neoplasms of the thyroid are most commonly derived from the epithelial elements of the gland and are divided into benign neoplasms (adenomas) and malignant neoplasms (carcinomas). The adenomas are subdivided descriptively into many entities, usually on the basis of the similarity of the neoplasm to variants of normal or abnormal thyroid architecture: macrofollicular, microfollicular, mixed macrofollicular and microfollicular, fetal, embryonal, or Hürthle cell. In addition, the term *atypical adenoma* is used to denote a benign-appearing follicular neoplasm (lacking invasive characteristics) that shows atypical cytologic features—for example, nuclei may be enlarged and hyperchromatic with pleomorphic features, suggestive of malignancy by classic cytologic criteria.

The primary carcinomas of the thyroid are divided into four main categories: papillary, follicular, medullary, and anaplastic. Papillary carcinoma is by far the most common, constituting about 90% of new thyroid malignancies at my institution. This disease is seen predominately in younger adults, although it can occur at almost any age. Generally, it is an indolent process with a tendency for local extension and spread to regional lymph nodes. Follicular and medullary carcinomas are intermediate in terms of aggressiveness. These tumors may occur at any age but are most frequently diagnosed in the adult years. Follicular carcinoma has a tendency

to metastasize via the bloodstream and may present with distant metastasis from an occult primary lesion. Medullary carcinoma is a malignant process involving the C cells of the thyroid, that is, the calcitonin-producing neuroendocrine cells of the gland. Medullary carcinoma is sometimes associated with multiple endocrine neoplasia but most frequently occurs in a nonfamilial sporadic form.[1]

Anaplastic carcinoma is a fairly unusual high-grade neoplasm occurring mainly in older persons and presenting as a rapidly growing neck mass with pain and obstructive symptoms. This is a highly virulent form of cancer, and most patients are dead within 1 year of diagnosis.[2-4] Unusual malignant conditions involving the thyroid include metastatic carcinoma, lymphoma, and sarcoma.

CYTOPATHOLOGIC DIAGNOSIS

Nonthyroid Cells

Several nonthyroid cell types may be seen in aspirates as "contaminant" cells from surrounding structures. The most frequent are fragments of fat or striate muscle from the tissues anterior to the thyroid. Occasionally, fragments of skin introduced into the needle during insertion are seen. Rarely, fragments of cartilage are seen—presumably obtained from thyroid cartilage or tracheal rings lying immediately behind the thyroid gland. Not infrequently, ciliated columnar epithelium is seen, again presumably from the trachea. (Congenital cysts—thyroglossal duct cysts or branchial cleft cysts—sometimes are lined by ciliated columnar epithelium or squamous epithelium; such cells may have diagnostic significance if obtained from a cyst.) Rarely, hematopoietic cells, including megakaryocytes, are observed. These cells are obtained when the needle enters the laryngeal or tracheal cartilage and aspirates cells from the bone marrow, where they are present during normal adult life.[5]

Benign Thyroid Nodule

Benign thyroid nodule (Fig. 5-1) is a term used to describe a cytologic picture compatible with a benign noninflammatory thyroid process. The cytologic findings are similar in an aspirate taken from a completely normal gland (an unlikely event), from a macrofollicular adenoma, or from a multinodular goiter. Thus, correlation of the cytologic picture with the clinical findings is important.

At low power, the benign nodule shows normal cellularity, generally with the presence of colloid and often some evidence of degeneration. Normal cellularity is difficult to define but is an impression garnered by examination of all the slides in a case rather than of a specific

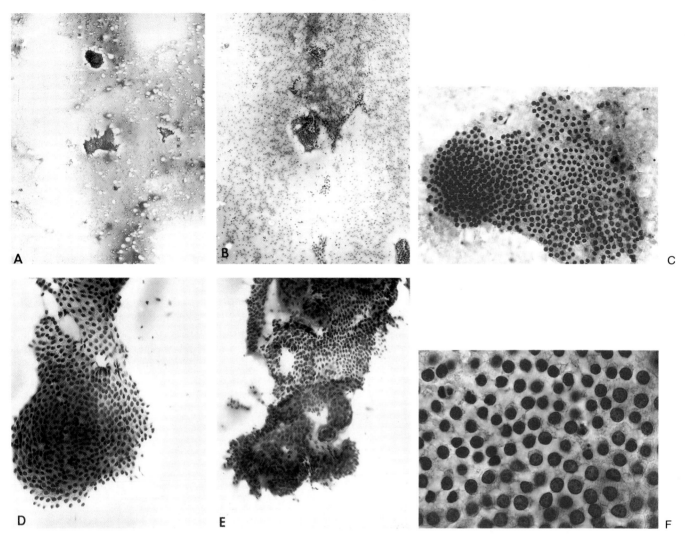

FIG. 5-1. Colloid nodule (benign thyroid nodule). **(A)** Scanning-power view. Background shows colloid with a few erythrocytes. Thyroid epithelial cells are present in cohesive sheets and clusters. (Papanicolaou stain, ×64) **(B)** Higher magnification shows cells distributed predominantly in cohesive sheets. At this magnification, the nuclear regularity first can be appreciated. (Papanicolaou stain, ×100) **(C)** Sheet of regular cells with uniform spacing, small round nuclei. (Papanicolaou stain, ×250) **(D)** High-power view reveals ill-defined cytoplasmic borders, although in some areas a hexagonal pattern is visible. Nuclei are round to oval and regular in size and staining characteristics. (Papanicolaou stain, ×250) **(E)** Follicular architecture is present in a microbiopsy fragment. These three-dimensional spheres may appear to contain colloid when appropriate focus is obtained. Observe the relative nuclear uniformity. (Papanicolaou stain, ×160) **(F)** High-power view. Nuclei are small, round, and regular, and their finely granular chromatin with small chromocenters is visible. (Papanicolaou stain, ×640)

microscopic field. The amount of epithelium may vary, but in the usual situation (with a 10× objective) one expects to see one or two aggregates of epithelial cells in a field. A field completely filled with cells at this magnification raises the question of hypercellularity, particularly if seen in multiple fields. In addition to the overall numbers of cells, the distribution of the cells—the low-power architecture—is important. In benign thyroid nodules, the cells generally are in sheets, sometimes are in small syncytia, and sometimes, in microbiopsy specimens, show the three-dimensional spherical architecture

of the thyroid follicle. Colloid is often present, appearing on the slide as a diffuse fluid material, often with bubbles, cracking, or erythrocytes within it. Colloid is sticky, like gelatin, and tends to show radial spiculations to cell groups and tissue fragments lying within it. In some situations, the colloid is more solid than fluid, and fairly discrete masses of amorphous, smooth, hyaline material are present; these usually stain green to pink in Papanicolaou preparations. Not infrequently, when follicular spheres are present, colloid can be seen centrally within this sphere.

At high magnification, the cells of benign thyroid nodules show a relatively regular pattern. They tend to be evenly spaced and orderly, although there may be some overlapping, depending on folding of sheets of epithelium or the thickness or depth of the microbiopsy material. The cytoplasm is scanty. Cell borders occasionally may be seen, but they often are ill defined. When present, the cell borders appear hexagonal, similar to the pattern seen in end-on views of endocervical cells. The nuclei normally are round and regular. Normal thyroid nuclei are 12 to 15 μm in diameter, about 1.5 times the size of an erythrocyte. The chromatin normally is evenly dispersed and finely granular, a feature often referred to as a "salt-and-pepper pattern." Nucleoli normally are either invisible or very small.

Completely normal cells show a uniform picture, although degenerative changes, which are common in the thyroid, may lead to a mild to moderate degree of pleomorphism. With aging, thyroid cells become somewhat more pleomorphic, which is reflected in aspirated material.

In microbiopsy fragments, spindle cell (stromal) elements are commonly seen surrounding follicular spheres or adjacent to sheets of epithelial cells. These stromal elements include endothelial cells, fibroblasts, and their associated collagenous stroma. Even a normal thyroid contains some foam cells in the colloid of follicular spaces, and thus the presence of a few foam cells is not considered remarkable.

Large numbers of foam cells indicate a degenerative phenomenon, most frequently cystic degeneration or hemorrhage with macrophage accumulation. If large numbers of foam cells are present, comments concerning evidence of degeneration are appropriate in addition to the main diagnosis of colloid nodule. Foam cells also may be present in malignant disease. Thus, these cells are evidence only of degeneration and do not indicate the nature of the underlying lesion.

A minimal number of thyroid epithelial cells should be present before a diagnosis of negative for malignancy is rendered. At my institution, the rule of six groups of well-preserved, benign-appearing cells has been adopted. The minimal number of cells per group is 12 to 15. If a very large sheet or a microbiopsy specimen containing several macrofollicles is seen, these units alone would meet the criterion for an adequate specimen. Whether one accepts the above definition of adequacy or chooses to be more stringent, it is important to keep in mind the

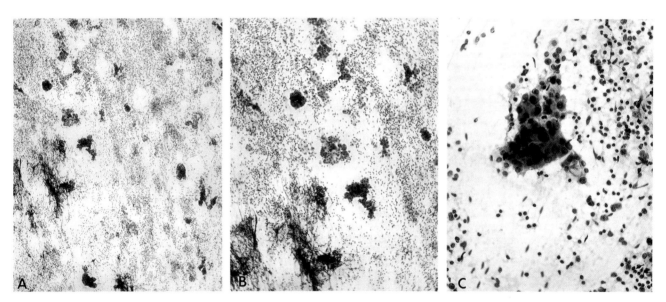

FIG. 5-2. Hashimoto's thyroiditis. **(A)** Scanning-power view. Observe the hypercellularity with a dispersed cell pattern. Cohesive epithelial groups are visible. Background is filled with lymphoid element. Some "squish" artifact is also present. (Papanicolaou stain, ×64) **(B)** Higher magnification shows bimorphic population of lymphocytes and Hürthle cells. (Papanicolaou stain, ×100) **(C)** High-power view. Centrally located is a group of Hürthle cells with abundant, finely granular cytoplasm and mild nuclear atypia. There is a mixed lymphoid inflammatory infiltrate in the background. (Papanicolaou stain, ×300) **(D)** Hürthle cells and accompanying lymphocytes. Observe the finely granular cytoplasm of Hürthle cells and their nuclear pleomorphism with prominent central nucleoli. (Papanicolaou stain, ×400) **(E)** Medium-power view of Hashimoto's thyroiditis showing lymphocytic inflammatory cell population in the background with irregular aggregates of Hürthle cell epithelial elements. (Papanicolaou stain, ×300) **(F)** Hashimoto's thyroiditis with atypical Hürthle cells. Multinucleation and pleomorphic nuclei with some prominent nucleoli are not uncommon in this condition. (Papanicolaou stain, ×640)

(continued)

need for adequate sampling. A diagnosis of negative based on inadequate material may turn out to be a false-negative result on subsequent tissue examination.

Hyperthyroidism

Hyperthyroidism usually is diagnosed clinically by features such as nervousness, tachycardia, heat intolerance, and easy sweating. The thyroid often is diffusely enlarged. The clinical impression generally is confirmed by increased concentrations of serum thyroid hormone. Fine needle aspiration is done only infrequently in this disease.

Aspirates from the hyperactive thyroid gland show increased cellularity and decreased colloid as a result of the rapid turnover of hormone. Smears are often hemorrhagic as a result of increased blood flow to the hyperactive gland. At my institution, limited experience with this entity has shown generalized enlargement of the epithelial cells and some increase in the amount of cytoplasm. Mild nuclear pleomorphism is present.[6,7]

Thyroiditis

Hashimoto's Thyroiditis

Hashimoto's thyroiditis (Fig. 5-2) is considered to be an autoimmune disease that is manifested histologically by chronic lymphocytic inflammation, Hürthle cell metaplasia, and progressive fibrosis. This disease is relatively common in the United States. It often presents as a diffuse goiter, sometimes slightly nodular. Cytologically, the findings are dominated by the presence of lymphocytes and Hürthle cell variants of thyroid epithelial cells. The relative amounts of these two cell populations vary depending on the stage of the disease process.[8-11]

Hürthle cells are epithelial lining cells that have become larger than normal because of an increase in their cytoplasm. The cytoplasm stains eosinophilic in histologic preparations, and electron microscopy shows large numbers of mitochondria. In Papanicolaou-stained material, the abundant cytoplasm has a very fine granularity, but the color may vary from pink to green to yellow-

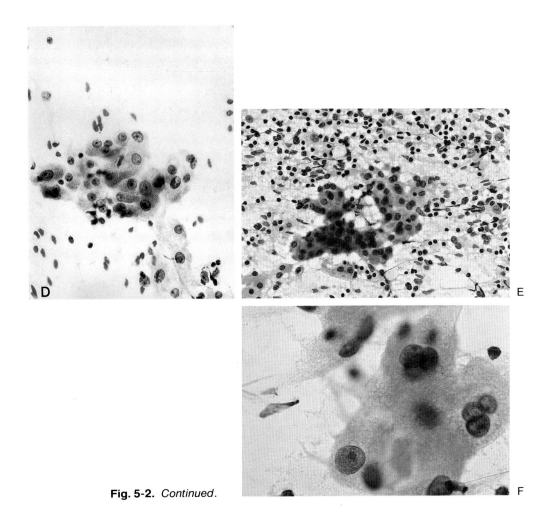

Fig. 5-2. *Continued.*

brown. Nuclei are larger than normal, often have prominent nucleoli, and may show a mild degree of grooving. Hürthle cells often are atypical and pleomorphic in Hashimoto's thyroiditis. The degree of Hürthle cell change is variable: well-developed cases are seen most frequently, but in a few cases relatively normal-appearing cells are present and only some cells show the Hürthle cell change.

As the disease progresses, the intensity of the lymphoid infiltrate decreases and the relative amount of fibrosis of the gland increases. In late stages of Hashimoto's thyroiditis, the aspirate may contain only a scanty number of cells because the gland is largely fibrotic. Hürthle cells may be obtained from the residual epithelial elements, and small numbers of lymphoid cells would be expected. Because the gland is being damaged by the inflammatory infiltrate, the amount of colloid present is generally scanty and often absent.

Careful examination of the character of the lymphoid inflammation is important. The possibility of lymphoma always must be considered. The lymphocytic cells should be predominantly mature lymphocytes associated with smaller numbers of immature lymphocytes, plasma cells, and histiocytic phagocytic cells. Tingible-body macrophages are common in Hashimoto's thyroiditis, but their presence does not entirely rule out the possibility of a malignant lesion. Histiocytic, multinucleated giant cells are not unusual in Hashimoto's thyroiditis. Usually, they are small to moderate in size and contain 4 to 10 nuclei; on occasion, they are larger and more prominent. The phenomenon of nuclear streak artifact (also referred to as "squish" artifact or lymphoid nest) is common in Hashimoto's thyroiditis. These areas of distorted, elongated nuclear material are due to fragility of the lymphoid nuclei and give the appearance of a tangled web. This streaking can occur with other cells as well, but it is most frequent with lymphocytes and thus with Hashimoto's thyroiditis.

The cytologic impression of Hashimoto's thyroiditis can be confirmed by the presence of antibodies to thyroglobulin and thyroid microsomes in the serum. In difficult cases, such serologic studies may be of value, but for most cases they probably are not necessary if the cytologic picture is clearcut.[12]

Subacute Thyroiditis (de Quervain's Thyroiditis, Granulomatous Thyroiditis)

Histologically, granulomatous inflammation is present with prominent, multinucleated giant cells. Cytologically (Fig. 5-3), subacute thyroiditis is recognized by the presence of large, multinucleated, histiocytic giant cells. These cells contain 50 to 100 uniform nuclei, and the cytoplasm of these cells is syncytial and does not contain phagocytized material. The aspirate otherwise shows de-

creased amounts of colloid, a mixed inflammatory infiltrate (often containing a modest number of neutrophils), epithelioid cells, and epithelial cells that show reactive changes (such as mild but uniform nuclear enlargement and some prominence of nucleoli). The Hürthle cell metaplasia of Hashimoto's thyroiditis is absent in subacute thyroiditis.[9]

Riedel's Fibrous Thyroiditis

Riedel's fibrous thyroiditis is an extremely rare disease. At my institution, there is no experience in diagnosing this disease cytologically. It is suspected that aspirates from Riedel's thyroiditis usually would be nondiagnostic, showing very few thyroid epithelial cells and perhaps some benign-appearing lymphocytes.

Neutrophilic Thyroiditis (Abscess)

Neutrophilic thyroiditis also is a rare disease. On occasion, an abscess can develop, often due to trauma and sometimes postoperatively. In these circumstances, abundant neutrophilic inflammation is present, indicative of abscess or acute inflammation. Neutrophilic inflammation sometimes is very prominent in anaplastic carcinoma, and a careful search should be made for a small population of high-grade carcinoma cells that may be obscured by excessive neutrophilic inflammation. Of course, abscesses or inflammatory processes of tissues adjacent to the thyroid (including lymph nodes) are not infrequent and must be considered.

Primary Neoplasms

Papillary Carcinoma

In my practice, papillary carcinoma is the most common primary malignancy of the thyroid. The cytologic features (Fig. 5-4) of this neoplasm are sufficiently clearcut that many cases can be diagnosed with confidence.[13,14] Because of limitations in sampling, degenerative changes, or unusual tumor variants, some cases are more difficult to diagnose, making a suspicious report appropriate.

At low power, the cells from papillary carcinoma often are arranged in papillary groups. These sometimes are narrow and frond shaped but are frequently thick and broad. A fibrovascular stromal core may be identified centrally, with tumor cells arranged on the periphery of this core. Frequently, the columnar neoplastic cells are arranged in an orderly perpendicular fashion, producing a straight, sharp edge of the papillary cell group. Some papillary carcinomas do not show papillary cell groups

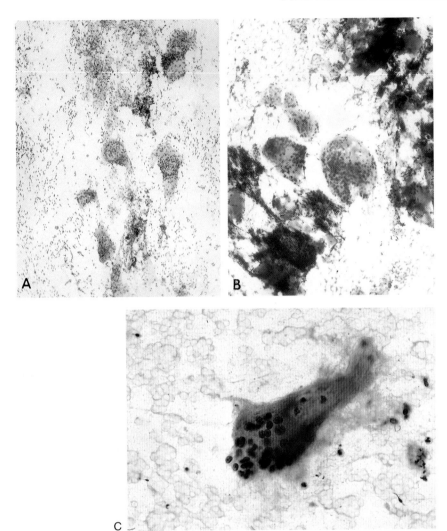

FIG. 5-3. Subacute thyroiditis. **(A)** Note the large number of multinucleated giant cells. Each giant cell contains more than 20 nuclei. There is some mixed inflammation associated with the giant cells. (Papanicolaou stain, ×100) **(B)** Observe the large number of bland histiocytic-type nuclei in these giant cells and the associated mixed inflammation with some "squish" artifact. (Papanicolaou stain, ×160) **(C)** Histiocytic multinucleated giant cells in subacute thyroiditis. Many nuclei, abundant syncytial cytoplasm, and a lack of phagocytized cytoplasmic debris are all expected in this condition. (Papanicolaou stain, ×300)

at low magnification, and thus their absence does not exclude the diagnosis.

Another arrangement of papillary carcinoma cells commonly seen at low magnification is monolayer sheets. This feature has limited use, however, because benign cells often are present in monolayer sheets also. Nuclear characteristics play a more important part in determining the nature of the cells than does the architectural arrangement in this situation. Some papillary carcinomas show a follicular growth pattern histologically; this may lead to a cytologic picture suggestive of follicular neoplasm at low magnification. However, the peculiar nuclear characteristics of papillary carcinoma usually can be appreciated even in these cases.

The cells of papillary carcinoma usually are larger than normal, contain more cytoplasm, and have a larger nucleus. Cell membranes tend to be well defined, and on occasion squamous differentiation is detectable, reflecting histologic squamous metaplasia. The nuclei are oval rather than round, often somewhat angulated with cor-

ners, and molded against each other, and the nuclear membrane tends to be irregular. Nuclei frequently overlap each other. The chromatin quality in papillary carcinoma is one of the most crucial cytologic features. Tumor cell nuclei are pale-staining and show less chromatin granularity than normal. These nuclei have been described as ground glass in appearance. This feature is variable, depending on the tumor as well as on fixation and staining factors. In many cases, the nuclear changes are evident; in others, there is a barely discernible alteration from normal. Longitudinal grooving of the nuclear membrane is another useful cytologic finding in papillary carcinoma. The grooves often impart a coffee bean appearance; from other angles, they may cause a notched appearance at the edge of the nucleus.

Intranuclear holes—actually, cytoplasmic intranuclear invagination—also are strongly suggestive of papillary carcinoma. Such holes need to be differentiated from artifactual bubbles or vacuolation. They should be reasonably large and have a crisp rim of nuclear mem-

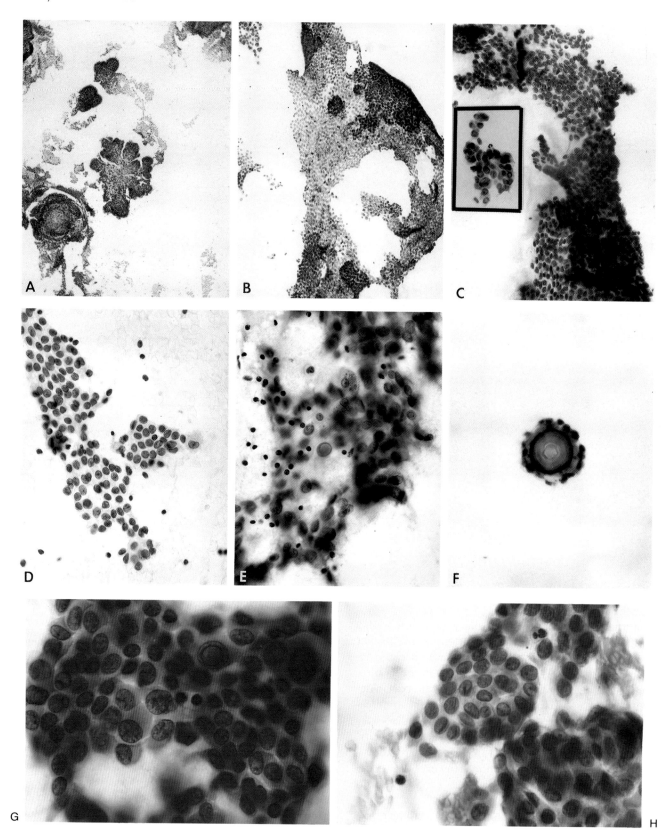

FIG. 5-4.

brane and chromatin material. Sometimes the holes are multiple, and often they are of different sizes. Occasionally, the hole largely replaces the nucleus, leaving only a thin rim of nuclear membrane peripherally.

Neither intranuclear holes nor grooving of the nuclear membrane is specific for papillary carcinoma. Grooving can occur in several situations, notably Hashimoto's thyroiditis, in which the Hürthle cells may show a mild degree of nuclear grooving. Intranuclear holes are common in papillary carcinoma but also are present in medullary carcinoma of the thyroid and have been reported, although rarely, in other benign and malignant conditions of the thyroid. Intranuclear holes are found in paragangliomas, which may mimic thyroid tumors clinically. In addition, hyalinizing trabecular adenoma (see later) shows the nuclear features described for papillary carcinoma—that is, enlarged, pale nuclei with intranuclear holes and grooving of the nuclear membrane.

Noncellular features may be useful in the diagnosis of papillary carcinoma. The colloid tends to be more solid than normal and sometimes shows a viscous or sticky quality. The viscous stretched colloid has been referred to as "bubble gum colloid" and, although rare, can be a useful diagnostic feature. Psammoma bodies are present in perhaps 10% to 20% of cases and are a useful diagnostic finding when present. On occasion, psammoma bodies may be one of a few diagnostic features present, such as in cystically degenerated papillary tumors.[15] At my institution, psammoma bodies are considered highly suggestive of papillary carcinoma, although they may be found, in rare cases, in association with other tumors or even in benign thyroid tissue.

Multinucleated histiocytic giant cells are often found in papillary carcinoma. Histologically, these cells frequently fill small extracellular spaces in association with colloid. Their presence cytologically is nonspecific; these cells also may be present in simple degeneration, in Hashimoto's thyroiditis, and (in large numbers and in large size) in subacute thyroiditis.

Rarely, a Hürthle cell variant of papillary carcinoma is encountered.[16] Cytologically, features consistent with Hürthle cell neoplasm (see later) are expected. In my experience, the nuclei generally resemble Hürthle cell tumors more than classic papillary carcinomas.

Follicular Neoplasms

Aspiration cytology has limitations in the definition of follicular neoplasms (Fig. 5-5). The histologic diagnosis of malignancy in follicular tumors is based on invasion of either the capsule or blood vessels.[17,18] Aspirated cells can indicate the presence of a cellular follicular neoplasm, but it is impossible to predict the presence or absence of invasive characteristics. Therefore, at my institution, all such neoplasms are considered potentially malignant and operation is recommended in most of these cases.[19]

The cardinal cytologic features of follicular neoplasm are hypercellularity, dispersed microfollicular pattern, and relative decrease in the amount of colloid present. Hypercellularity must be judged in specific fields and for the overall specimen. It is possible for a macrofollicular benign nodule to produce some hypercellular zones. Even in these zones, however, the cells tend to show either a macrofollicular architecture or are present in sheets or other aggregates.

The aspirate from a follicular neoplasm has a microfollicular pattern. The follicles usually are composed of 6 to 12 nuclei surrounding a small central lumen. Colloid may be present in the lumen but often is absent. These microfollicular rings are dispersed rather than in cohesive groups or sheets, producing fields containing largely separate microfollicular units. Some of the rings are easier to see than others. The amount of colloid present is variable but generally decreased compared with the number of cells present. Nuclear atypia may be present. When present, it often is mild. On occasion, there is appreciable nuclear enlargement, pleomorphism, and prominence of nucleoli. It is unusual to see markedly pleomorphic cells or necrosis in follicular neoplasms.

FIG. 5-4. Papillary carcinoma. (A) Low-power view. Tumor cells are arranged in papillary configurations and in some flat sheets. A small amount of stroma tissue (fibroblasts and blood vessels) is present centrally in papillary fronds. (Papanicolaou stain, ×100) (B) Sheet of tumor cells. These cells tend to be arranged in flat sheets. (Papanicolaou stain, ×160) (C) High-power view. Nuclei are enlarged and contain pale chromatin. Small nucleoli are present. Longitudinal grooving of nuclear membrane is also present. (Papanicolaou stain, ×250) Grooving of nuclear membrane (inset). (Papanicolaou stain, ×400) (D) High-power magnification view showing pale, diffuse chromatin and nuclear grooving and notching. (Papanicolaou stain, ×400) (E) Intranuclear holes in aspirated cells. Observe the size of the holes in relation to the nuclei and their smooth, sharp rim of nuclear membrane. (Papanicolaou stain, ×400) (F) Psammoma body with concentric laminations and surrounding tumor cells in an aspirate from a cystic thyroid nodule. On pathologic examination, the lesion proved to be a cystically degenerated papillary carcinoma. (Papanicolaou stain, ×400) (G) Cells of papillary carcinoma with large, oval, and irregular nuclei showing pale chromatin pattern and an intranuclear hole. Cytoplasm is abundant. (Papanicolaou stain, ×640) (H) Cells of papillary carcinoma—large oval nuclei with flattened sides and crowding, pale chromatin, and grooving of the nuclear membrane. (Papanicolaou stain, ×540)

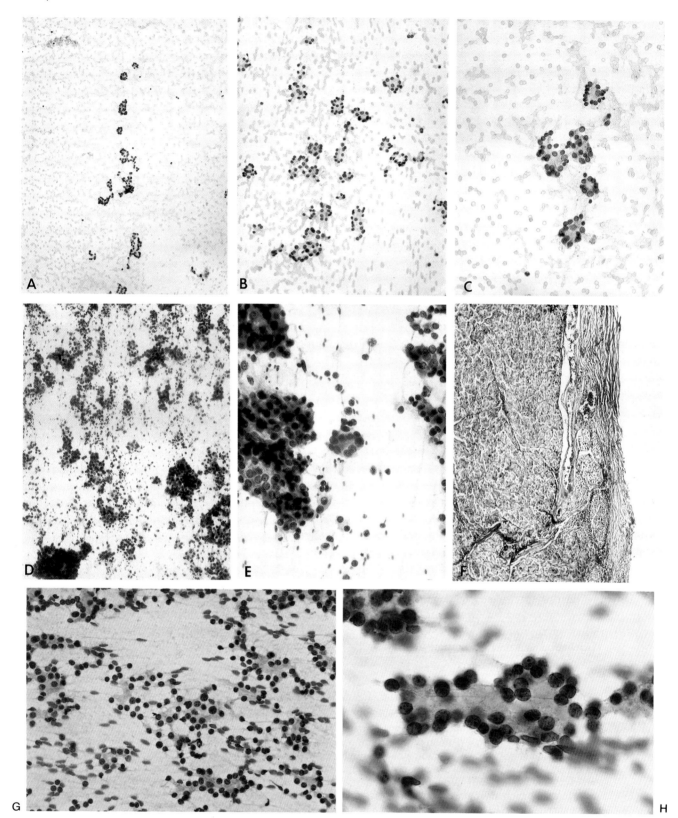

FIG. 5-5.

A gray zone exists between the benign aspirate that is somewhat cellular and the minimal findings sufficient for a diagnosis of follicular neoplasm. Precise delineation of this zone is not possible, and each case must be evaluated on the basis of the quantity and quality of the cells present. Also, the cytologic evaluation should be integrated with the clinical impression. In my experience, the risk of malignancy subsequent to the cytologic diagnosis of follicular neoplasm is considerably greater in a single isolated thyroid nodule than in a multinodular gland. In addition, cases can show a greater or lesser degree of cytologic abnormality that loosely correlates with the risk of subsequent malignancy.[20,21]

Because of the limitations of aspiration cytology in predicting malignancy by light microscopy, a number of investigators have examined ancillary techniques. Quantitative microscopy has been used to assess nuclear size (perimeter or diameter) or degree of nuclear roundness in an attempt to discriminate between benign and malignant lesions. Although initial results were promising, subsequent analysis has proved the limited value of this approach because these features overlap considerably in the benign and malignant groups.[22] Similarly, analysis of DNA content by static image analysis or by flow cytometry is not diagnostic of malignancy because of overlap of the DNA patterns in benign and malignant neoplasms.[23]

There is no way of accurately predicting the subsequent histologic diagnosis, and all such neoplasms should be removed if clinically indicated. In our hands, about 15% of the cases with a cytologic diagnosis of follicular neoplasm have proved to be carcinoma on pathologic examination of the surgical specimen. Ninety-five percent of these cases prove to be neoplasms, but they most frequently are adenomas rather than follicular carcinomas.

Hyalinizing trabecular adenoma[24,25] is considered a special subgroup of follicular neoplasm. Histologically, this lesion shows spindle-shaped cells arranged in nests and trabecular cords with various degrees of hyaline fibrosis and cystic change. This lesion frequently contains psammoma bodies, and it is encapsulated and not invasive. These cells stain for thyroglobulin by immunoper-

oxidase techniques and are negative for thyrocalcitonin. Cytologic features include spindle-shaped cells with enlarged nuclei that show pale, "washed-out" chromatin, grooving of the nuclear membrane, and intranuclear holes. The cytologic picture may be confused with either papillary carcinoma or medullary carcinoma.[26]

Hürthle Cell Neoplasms

Most, but not all, Hürthle cell lesions are variants of follicular neoplasm. As such, the histologic diagnosis of Hürthle cell adenoma or carcinoma depends on the presence or absence of capsular or vascular invasion.[27] The cytologic method cannot evaluate invasiveness, and therefore Hürthle cell neoplasms as a group must be considered suspicious for malignancy. The cytologic pattern (Fig. 5-6) is characterized by hypercellularity, a relatively pure population of Hürthle cells, decreased colloid, and a variable degree of cytologic atypia.[28,29] Some cases show tremendous hypercellularity with considerable nuclear atypia and absence of colloid and are clearly abnormal. There is a borderline category, however, with minimal deviations from what is considered normal. Some aspirates from benign lesions show a few Hürthle cells, but this is not automatically a suspicious cytologic result. The overall degree of cellularity, the proportion of the cells present that are Hürthle cells, the amount of colloid, the architectural pattern, and the degree of cytologic atypia all play a role in the cytologic evaluation.

One of the most important cytologic differential diagnoses with Hürthle cell neoplasm is Hashimoto's thyroiditis. A careful search should be made for a lymphoid inflammatory component in the aspirate. A relatively small number of lymphocytes may be significant, indicating Hashimoto's thyroiditis rather than a true Hürthle cell neoplasm. In some patients with Hashimoto's thyroiditis, hyperplastic Hürthle cell nodules develop but probably are not true neoplasms: they lack a capsule and do not compress adjacent tissue. An aspirate from such a nodule has cytologic features indistinguishable from those of Hürthle cell neoplasm.

FIG. 5-5. Follicular neoplasm. **(A)** Low-power view. Cells are distributed in microfollicular rings with scanty colloid. Rings are dispersed in noncohesive fashion. (Papanicolaou stain, ×100) **(B)** Mild nuclear variability is detected, but the primary diagnostic feature is the dispersed microfollicular rings (small amounts of colloid may be present within these rings). (Papanicolaou stain, ×160) **(C)** High-power view shows microfollicular rings and mild degree of nuclear pleomorphism. At operation, this lesion proved to be follicular carcinoma. (Papanicolaou stain, ×250) **(D)** Specimen is markedly hypercellular with poor cell cohesion. Minimal evidence of follicular architecture is present. (Papanicolaou stain, ×160) **(E)** At high magnification, generalized nuclear enlargement, poor cohesion, and a single microfollicular ring. (Papanicolaou stain, ×400) **(F)** Invasion of tumor cells into a blood vessel. (Hematoxylin–eosin stain, ×100) **(G)** Medium-power view from follicular neoplasm showing dispersed microfollicular pattern and hypercellularity. (Papanicolaou stain, ×250) **(H)** High-power view of follicular neoplasm showing microfollicles. Individual nuclear atypia is not particularly impressive (surgery subsequently showed a follicular adenoma). (Papanicolaou stain, ×540)

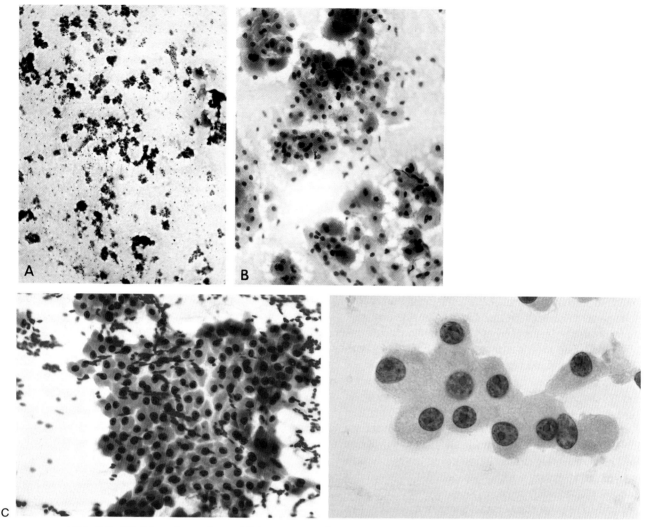

FIG. 5-6. Hürthle cell neoplasm. **(A)** Low-power view shows hypercellularity, poor cell cohesion, and relative lack of colloid. (Papanicolaou stain, ×100) **(B)** Higher magnification shows abundant cytoplasm that is finely granular. There is a mild degree of nuclear pleomorphism. (Papanicolaou stain, ×300) **(C)** Cells from Hürthle cell neoplasm showing a relatively cohesive group of epithelial cells—purely Hürthle cell type. No lymphocytic inflammation is identified. Colloid is absent. (Papanicolaou stain, ×400) **(D)** High-power view of follicular neoplasm shows atypical Hürthle cells with somewhat variable nuclei, coarse chromatin, and prominent nucleoli. (Papanicolaou stain, ×640)

If the clinical suspicion is Hashimoto's thyroiditis or if the cytologic features point toward that possibility, further diagnostic efforts can be considered. First, other areas can be aspirated in an attempt to establish the diagnosis of Hashimoto's thyroiditis. Second, studies for serum antithyroid antibodies can be performed. It is possible for a Hürthle cell neoplasm and even a Hürthle cell carcinoma to develop in a patient with Hashimoto's thyroiditis. The presence of thyroiditis lends only relative security to a negative diagnosis when Hürthle cell neoplasm is suspected, and it does not completely negate the cytologic observations and clinical circumstances.

In our experience, the diagnosis of Hürthle cell neo-plasm is slightly less reliable than that of follicular neoplasm. On subsequent tissue examination, 85% of cases prove to be neoplastic; the rest usually show either thyroiditis or multinodular goiter with Hürthle cell features. As with follicular neoplasms, 15% of cases show malignancy at operation after the cytologic diagnosis of Hürthle cell neoplasm. Also as with follicular neoplasms, special studies of the aspirate for cell morphology or DNA content by flow cytometry are imprecise predictors of malignancy.[30,31]

A small number of lesions diagnosed cytologically as Hürthle cell neoplasms prove to be papillary tumors on histologic examination. At my institution, prediction of papillary carcinomas of the Hürthle cell type has not been possible cytologically, and such cases have simply been classified as Hürthle cell neoplasms.

Medullary Carcinoma

Medullary carcinoma (Fig. 5-7) is a malignant tumor that differentiates toward C cells (thyrocalcitonin-producing cells) of the normal thyroid gland. These tumors are unusual—our total experience is about 40 cases.

Medullary carcinoma is a protean neoplasm with several histologic variants.[1] Similarly, the cytologic picture is variable.[32-35] The most common presentation is a hypercellular aspirate with poor cell cohesion and bipolar, spindle-shaped cells. The cytoplasm is slight to moderate in amount and reasonably well defined in most cases. The nuclei show significant atypia, although this may be subtle and focal, and a search may be necessary to identify the atypical areas. The nuclei show the coarse chromatin clumping of neuroendocrine tumors, similar to a carcinoid tumor (in many but not all instances). Multinucleation is common. Intranuclear holes are seen in

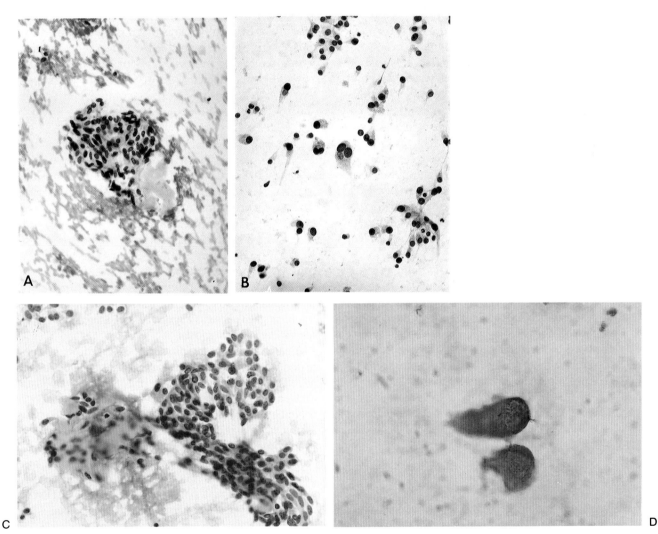

FIG. 5-7. Medullary carcinoma of the thyroid. **(A)** Tumor cells and amyloid. Cytoplasm is poorly defined, but there is a tendency toward elongated spindle forms. (Papanicolaou stain, ×300) **(B)** Note the dispersed, noncohesive cell pattern and tendency toward elongated cytoplasmic forms. Nuclei tend to be eccentric, and some multinucleation is present. (Papanicolaou stain, ×300) **(C)** Medium-power view of cells and amyloid material from medullary carcinoma. These cells are spindled and elongated and are associated with green-staining amyloid. (Papanicolaou stain, ×300) **(D)** Immunoperoxidase stain for thyrocalcitonin on cells from medullary carcinoma (previously alcohol fixed and Papanicolaou stained). Positivity of the cytoplasm and morphology of the cells are good evidence for medullary carcinoma. (×640)

many medullary carcinomas, but, in contrast to papillary carcinoma, the nuclei show hyperchromasia rather than the pale, washed-out chromatin of papillary tumors. There is no particular tendency toward grooving of the nuclear membrane, in contrast to papillary carcinoma or hyalinizing trabecular adenoma.

When medullary carcinoma is suspected, amyloid may be found in association with the tumor cells. Amyloid appears as solid, rather irregular fragments of green-staining hyaline substance on Papanicolaou staining. There often are streaked nuclear remnants in the amyloid, which helps to distinguish it from colloid. Amyloid is difficult to separate from colloid by Papanicolaou stain, and an overstain by the Congo red method is very useful for confirming amyloid in suspected cases.

Some medullary carcinomas present a cytologic picture closely mimicking that of lymphoma or plasmacytoma. Such cases show minimal cell cohesion, producing a dispersed single-cell pattern mimicking a lymphoid neoplasm. In addition, the cytoplasm may be scanty and ill defined, and the nuclei tend to be eccentric. This feature, in combination with coarse chromatin clumping, produces a picture very similar to that of plasmacytic differentiation and may give the examiner the impression of a plasmacytoid lymphoma. However, careful examination discloses cells with too much cytoplasm for a lymphoid neoplasm, tending to show a bipolar, spindle cell configuration. In addition, the degree of pleomorphism and the multinucleation in medullary carcinoma help distinguish it from lymphoid neoplasm. Individual cases may be difficult.

A reliable immunostain for thyrocalcitonin is available, and this is very useful in confirming the diagnosis of medullary carcinoma in difficult cases. Typical cases showing the described cytologic features and demonstrating amyloid confirmed by a Congo red stain probably do not need to be confirmed with a thyrocalcitonin stain. However, some difficult cases can be resolved by using the immunocytochemical technique. Medullary carcinoma of the thyroid also produces carcinoembryonic antigen, and immunostaining for it also may be helpful.

Anaplastic Carcinoma

Aspirates from anaplastic carcinoma (Fig. 5-8) show cells with classic malignant cytologic characteristics.[36] Most often, the cells show extreme atypia with coarse chromatin, hyperchromasia, macronucleoli, marked nuclear pleomorphism, and mitotic activity, including atypical mitotic figures. In addition, necrosis is frequently observed, with pyknotic debris and cytoplasmic fragments associated with the viable tumor cells. Neutrophilic inflammation is common, and, in some cases, the necrosis and inflammation are predominant, obscuring

the tumor cells in the background. When abundant purulent inflammation is present in a thyroid aspirate, anaplastic carcinoma should be considered.

The three histologic subtypes of anaplastic carcinoma are giant cell, spindle cell, and small cell. Giant cell carcinoma is most frequent and shows cells similar to those in many other pleomorphic giant cell carcinomas. The spindle cell variant may produce a cytologic picture mimicking that of sarcoma, and the small cell variant shows a picture like that of small cell undifferentiated carcinoma of the lung. Differentiation of small cell carcinoma from lymphoma is important, and immunostains for epithelial and lymphoid markers or electron microscopy may be helpful in difficult cases.[37] A small number of anaplastic carcinomas of the thyroid show C-cell differentiation and thus are anaplastic variants of medullary carcinoma. This diagnosis would be difficult to determine on a Papanicolaou-stained preparation and would require an immunostain for confirmation. With regard to immunostains, only 25% to 30% of anaplastic carcinomas are positive for thyroglobulin, and a negative stain does not preclude the diagnosis.

Metastatic Carcinoma

Metastatic carcinoma (Fig. 5-9) should be considered in any case showing high-grade tumor cells or a pattern that does not exhibit the usual characteristics of papillary, follicular, or medullary carcinomas. High-grade carcinoma metastatic to the thyroid from other locations such as the breast or the lung can mimic a high-grade primary thyroid neoplasm.[38–40] Immunostaining may be helpful in this regard, but most anaplastic tumors of the thyroid are negative on immunostaining for thyroglobulin, so negative results cannot be considered definitive in the differential diagnosis.

A careful history and physical examination and appropriate laboratory and radiologic studies provide the most effective way to differentiate primary from metastatic malignancy. On occasion, this problem cannot be resolved cytologically or clinically, and open tissue biopsy is needed to make the distinction.

In some clinical circumstances, immunostaining for various markers may be useful in identifying the origin of disease metastatic to the thyroid. An example is malignant melanoma: a positive S-100 protein or HMB-45 immunostain may help confirm the cytologic and clinical impression of melanoma. Unfortunately, a large number of tumors have no specific markers, including the most common primary tumors that metastasize to the thyroid such as lung, kidney, and breast.

Lymphoma

Cytologic diagnosis of lymphoma involving the thyroid poses the same problem as lymphoma at any other

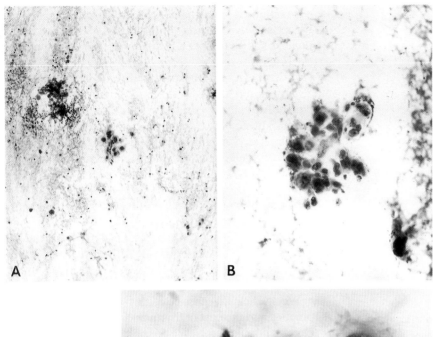

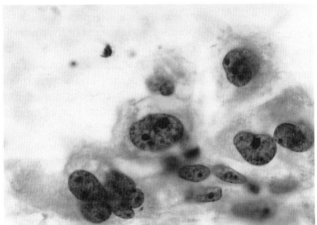

FIG. 5-8. Anaplastic carcinoma. **(A)** Low-power view shows large amount of necrosis and some inflammation; a few viable tumor cells are present in the background. (Papanicolaou stain, ×160) **(B)** At higher magnification, observe the marked pleomorphism and hyperchromasia of nuclei with prominent nucleoli. Necrotic debris is present at the periphery of this cell group. (Papanicolaou stain, ×400) **(C)** High-power view of anaplastic carcinoma cells showing marked nuclear pleomorphism, hyperchromasia, and very prominent nucleoli. Necrotic debris is present in the background. (Papanicolaou stain, ×300)

body site. Lymphoma in the thyroid may be a primary event, or it may be part of widespread systemic disease; therefore, the history may or may not be helpful. Primary lymphoma of the thyroid often presents as a slowly enlarging mass, sometimes with clinical or historic evidence of associated Hashimoto's thyroiditis.[41]

Cytologically, the monotony of lymphoma cells (Fig. 5-10) contrasts with the pleomorphic picture of benign lymphoid infiltrates such as Hashimoto's thyroiditis. The diagnosis is difficult, and it is easily overlooked on the assumption that the lymphoid cell population represents Hashimoto's thyroiditis. One needs to look carefully at the background lymphoid population for cytologic evidence of lymphoma in cases of Hashimoto's thyroiditis. The morphology of lymphoid cells is altered if there has been drying during preparation, and it is best to ignore cells that show air-drying artifact. (It is often useful to prepare a few air-dried slides stained with Diff-Quick or another Romanowsky method if there is a clinical suspicion of lymphoma.[10,42])

The practice at my institution is to confirm a cytologic diagnosis of lymphoma by biopsy so that part of the specimen can be used for frozen-section immunostaining and phenotyping. Some centers have reported success in using cytologic material for immunophenotyping, and this method may become more common in the future.

Nonthyroid Disease

A mass in the neck that from clinical studies is thought to be thyroidal may actually be an enlarged lymph node adjacent to the thyroid or some other nonthyroidal lesion. In my experience, many cases suspected to be thyroid neoplasm have turned out to be lymphoma or Hodgkin's disease involving adjacent lymph nodes. Paraganglioma may occur close enough to the thyroid to be clinically confusing. An aspirate shows poorly cohesive polygonal cells—nuclei show intranuclear holes.[43] Therefore, if the slides do not contain thyroid epithelial cells, nonthyroid abnormality should be considered.

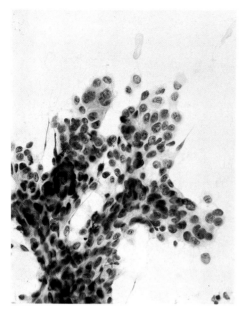

FIG. 5-9. Thyroid aspirate of lesion metastatic from a previous squamous cell carcinoma of the esophagus. Although clearly malignant, these cells do not show the usual patterns of primary thyroid carcinoma. In such situations, metastatic disease must be considered. (Papanicolaou stain, ×400)

Sarcomas

Sarcomatous involvement of the thyroid is extremely rare. At my institution, too few such cases have been seen to allow generalizations. If malignant-appearing cells are present that are poorly cohesive and generally bipolar or elongated, sarcoma is one of the considerations. Pleomorphic carcinoma or pseudomalignant processes such as fasciitis also should be considered.

COMMENT

Cytologic diagnosis should clearly categorize cases into one of four groups: negative for malignancy, suspicious for malignancy, positive for malignancy, and nondiagnostic. Within these categories, descriptive and histologic comments are used as indicated. In examination of more than 13,000 specimens at my institution, the distribution in these four categories has been as follows: negative, 65%; suspicious, 11%; positive, 4%; and nondiagnostic, 20%. These figures are similar to those of other series.[44]

Short of obtaining a tissue diagnosis in every case, it is impossible to ascertain the precise accuracy of aspiration cytologic study. The primary concern is the accurate identification of cases with malignant neoplasm. The bias in cytologic examination is to minimize false-negative reports at the expense of performing operation on a fair number of cases with benign disease. Through 1994 at my institution, satisfactory cytologic specimens were obtained from about 900 known malignancies, and the sensitivity rate was 97%—that is, 97% of the malignancies showed either a positive or suspicious cytologic picture.

A diagnosis of positive for malignancy has been made 525 times and has been confirmed either histologically or clinically in all but four cases (four false-positive reports, 0.8%). Thus, in my experience, a positive cytologic study almost always means malignancy is present. The suspicious for malignancy category includes the group of follicular and Hürthle cell neoplasms, which, as discussed, represent a limitation of the technique. Overall, about 30% of cytologically suspicious cases prove to be malignant when examined pathologically.

These comments apply only to satisfactory cytologic specimens. Several cases in which the cytologic features were nondiagnostic have proved to be malignant at operation.

We studied the impact of this procedure on thyroid practice and the cost of thyroid nodule evaluation in our patient population.[45] We found a decrease in the percentage of patients undergoing thyroid operation for possible malignancy and approximately a doubling of the yield of malignancy at surgical examination. We estimated that the total cost of medical care per patient decreased by about 25%.

CONCLUSIONS

Within reasonable expectations, aspiration cytologic study of the thyroid is an accurate and worthwhile diag-

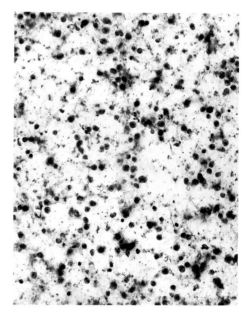

FIG. 5-10. High-power view of cells from thyroid lymphoma. Nuclei are moderately large and open and show some irregularities of outline. Cytoplasm is very scanty. Large amount of cytoplasmic and nuclear debris is present in the background. (Papanicolaou stain, ×400)

nostic tool.[46] Fine needle aspiration is more accurate than any other technique, short of operation, for determining the presence or absence of thyroid malignancy. In addition, it offers valuable information in many cases of benign disease. The central role of fine needle aspiration in the management of thyroid nodules has been extensively discussed[47-49]—my experience and that of my colleagues support this concept also. Fine needle aspiration of the thyroid does demand some interest and knowledge on the part of the cytopathologist. At my institution, a core group of interested clinicians and laboratorians has been established, and the concentration of experience in this group has improved performance and increased confidence in this technique.

REFERENCES

1. Uribe M, Fenoglio-Preiser CM, Grimes M, et al. Medullary carcinoma of the thyroid gland: clinical, pathological, and immunohistochemical features with review of the literature. Am J Surg Pathol 1985;9:577.
2. Carcangiu ML, Steeper T, Zampi G, et al. Anaplastic thyroid carcinoma: a study of 70 cases. Am J Clin Pathol 1985;83:135.
3. Nel CJ, van Heerden JA, Goellner JR, et al. Anaplastic carcinoma of the thyroid: a clinicopathologic study of 82 cases. Mayo Clin Proc 1985;60:51.
4. Shvero J, Gal R, Avidor I, et al. Anaplastic thyroid carcinoma: a clinical, histologic, and immunohistochemical study. Cancer 1988;62:319.
5. Gay JD, Bjornsson J, Goellner JR. Hematopoietic cells in thyroid fine-needle aspirates for cytologic study: report of two cases. Mayo Clin Proc 1985;60:123.
6. Jayaram G, Singh B, Marwaha RK. Grave's disease: appearance in cytologic smears from fine needle aspirates of the thyroid gland. Acta Cytol 1989;33:36.
7. Myren J, Sivertssen E. Thin-needle biopsy of the thyroid gland in the diagnosis of thyrotoxicosis. Acta Endocrinol (Copehn) 1962;39:431.
8. Friedman M, Shimaoka K, Rao U, et al. Diagnosis of chronic lymphocytic thyroiditis (nodular presentation) by needle aspiration. Acta Cytol 1981;25:513.
9. Guarda LA, Baskin HJ. Inflammatory and lymphoid lesions of the thyroid gland: cytopathology by fine-needle aspiration. Am J Clin Pathol 1987;87:14.
10. Kini SR, Miller JM, Hamburger JI. Problems in the cytologic diagnosis of the "cold" thyroid nodule in patients with lymphocytic thyroiditis. Acta Cytol 1981;25:506.
11. Ravinsky E, Safneck JR. Differentiation of Hashimoto's thyroiditis from thyroid neoplasms in fine needle aspirates. Acta Cytol 1988;32:854.
12. Baker BA, Gharib H, Markowitz H. Correlation of thyroid antibodies and cytologic features in suspected autoimmune thyroid disease. Am J Med 1983;74:941.
13. Kini SR, Miller JM, Hamburger JI, et al. Cytopathology of the papillary carcinoma of the thyroid by fine needle aspiration. Acta Cytol 1980;24:511.
14. Miller TR, Bottles K, Holly EA, et al. A step-wise logistic regression analysis of papillary carcinoma of the thyroid. Acta Cytol 1986;30:285.
15. Goellner JR, Johnson DA. Cytology of cystic papillary carcinoma of the thyroid. Acta Cytol 1982;26:797.
16. Hill JH, Werkhaven JA, DeMay RM. Hürthle cell variant of papillary carcinoma of the thyroid gland. Otolaryngol Head Neck Surg 1988;98:338.
17. Kahn NF, Perzin KH. Follicular carcinoma of the thyroid: an evaluation of the histologic criteria used for diagnosis. Pathol Annu 1983;18:221.
18. Lang W, Georgii A, Stauch G, et al. The differentiation of atypical

19. Gharib H, Goellner JR, Zinsmeister AR, et al. Fine-needle aspiration biopsy of the thyroid: the problem of suspicious cytologic findings. Ann Intern Med 1984;101:25.
20. Kini SR, Miller JM, Hamburger JI, et al. Cytopathology of follicular lesions of the thyroid gland. Diagn Cytopathol 1985;1:123.
21. Miller JM, Kini SR, Hamburger JI. The diagnosis of malignant follicular neoplasms of the thyroid by needle biopsy. Cancer 1985;55:2812.
22. Salmon I, Kiss R, Franc B, et al. Comparison of morphonuclear features in normal, benign and neoplastic thyroid tissue by digital cell image analysis. Anal Quant Cytol Histol 1992;14:47.
23. Oyama T, Vickery AL Jr, Preffer FI, et al. A comparative study of flow cytometry and histopathologic findings in thyroid follicular carcinomas and adenomas. Hum Pathol 1994;25:271.
24. Carney JA, Ryan J, Goellner JR. Hyalinizing trabecular adenoma of the thyroid gland. Am J Surg Pathol 1987;11:583.
25. Bronner MP, LiVolsi VA, Jennings TA. Paraganglioma-like adenomas of the thyroid. Surg Pathol 1988;1:383.
26. Goellner JR, Carney JA. Cytologic features of fine-needle aspirates of hyalinizing trabecular adenoma of the thyroid. Am J Clin Pathol 1989;91:115.
27. Bronner MS, LiVolsi VA. Oxyphilic (Ashanazy/Hürthle cell) tumors of the thyroid: microscopic features predict biologic behavior. Surg Pathol 1988;1:137.
28. Kini SR, Miller JM, Hamburger JI. Cytopathology of Hürthle cell lesions of the thyroid gland by fine needle aspiration. Acta Cytol 1981;25:647.
29. Mishriki YY, Lane BP, Lozowski MS, et al. Hürthle-cell tumor arising in the mediastinal ectopic thyroid and diagnosed by fine needle aspiration: light microscopic and ultrastructural features. Acta Cytol 1983;27;188.
30. Bondeson L, Bondeson AG, Lindholm K, et al. Morphometric studies on nuclei in smears of fine needle aspirates from oxyphilic tumors of the thyroid. Acta Cytol 1983;27:437.
31. McLeod MK, Thompson NW, Hudson JL, et al. Flow cytometric measurements of nuclear DNA and ploidy analysis in Hürthle cell neoplasms of the thyroid. Arch Surg 1988;123:849.
32. Bose S, Kapila K, Verma K. Medullary carcinoma of the thyroid: a cytological, immunocytochemical, and ultrastructural study. Diagn Cytopathol 1992;8:28.
33. Geddie WR, Bedard YC, Strawbridge HT. Medullary carcinoma of the thyroid in the fine-needle aspiration biopsies. Am J Clin Pathol 1984;82:552.
34. Collins BT, Cramer HM, Tabatowski K, et al. Fine needle aspiration of medullary carcinoma of the thyroid: cytomorphology, immunocytochemistry and electron microscopy. Acta Cytol 1995;39:920.
35. Kini SR, Miller JM, Hamburger JI, et al. Cytopathologic features of medullary carcinoma of the thyroid. Arch Pathol Lab Med 1984;108:156.
36. Schneider V, Frable WJ. Spindle and giant cell carcinoma of the thyroid: cytologic diagnosis by fine needle aspiration. Acta Cytol 1980;24:184.
37. Burt AD, Kerr DJ, Brown IL, et al. Lymphoid and epithelial markers in small cell anaplastic thyroid tumours. J Clin Pathol 1985;38:893.
38. Chacho MS, Greenebaum E, Moussouris HF, et al. Value of aspiration cytology of the thyroid in metastatic disease. Acta Cytol 1987;31:705.
39. Smith SA, Gharib H, Goellner JR. Fine-needle aspiration: usefulness for diagnosis and management of metastatic carcinoma to the thyroid. Arch Intern Med 1987;147:311.
40. Watts NB. Carcinoma metastatic to the thyroid: prevalence and diagnosis by fine-needle aspiration cytology. Am J Med Sci 1987;293:13.
41. Compagno J, Oertel JE. Malignant lymphoma and other lymphoproliferative disorders of the thyroid gland: a clinicopathologic study of 245 cases. Am J Clin Pathol 1980;74:1.
42. Matsuda M, Sone H, Koyama H, et al. Fine-needle aspiration cytology of malignant lymphoma of the thyroid. Diagn Cytopathol 1987;3:244.

adenomas and encapsulated follicular carcinomas in the thyroid gland. Virchows Arch A Pathol Anat Histopathol 1980;385:125.

43. González-Cámpora R, Otal-Salaverri C, Panea-Flores P, et al. Fine needle aspiration cytology of paraganglionic tumors. Acta Cytol 1988;32:386.

44. Gharib H, Goellner JR. Fine-needle aspiration biopsy of the thyroid: an appraisal. Ann Intern Med 1993;118:282.

45. Hamberger B, Gharib H, Melton LJ III, et al. Fine-needle aspiration biopsy of thyroid nodules: impact on thyroid practice and cost of care. Am J Med 1982;73:381.

46. Akerman M, Tennvall J, Biörklund A, et al. Sensitivity and specificity of fine needle aspiration cytology in the diagnosis of tumors of the thyroid gland. Acta Cytol 1985;29:850.

47. Bisi H, de Camargo RY, Longatto Filho A. Role of fine-needle aspiration cytology in the management of thyroid nodules: review of experience with 1,925 cases. Diagn Cytopathol 1992;8:504.

48. Mazzaferri EL. Management of a solitary thyroid nodule. N Engl J Med 1993;328:553.

49. Silverman JF, West RL, Larkin EW, et al. The role of fine-needle aspiration biopsy in the rapid diagnosis and management of thyroid neoplasm. Cancer 1986;57:1164.

Fine Needle Aspiration of Subcutaneous Organs and Masses,
edited by Yener S. Erozan and Thomas A. Bonfiglio.
Lippincott–Raven Publishers, Philadelphia, © 1996.

CHAPTER 6

Fine Needle Aspiration of the Salivary Glands

Ibrahim Ramzy and Dina R. Mody

NORMAL SALIVARY GLANDS

Salivary glands can be divided into major and minor glands. The major glands include the parotid, submandibular and sublingual glands. The minor glands are widely distributed under the mucosa of the oral cavity and the upper aerodigestive tract. Salivary glands are compound tubuloalveolar glands that are divided by fibrous septa into lobes and lobules. Each lobule is made up of secretory units called *acini* that drain into ducts. The acini are lined by epithelial and myoepithelial cells, which are surrounded by basement membrane. The parotid is a serous gland, and hence the acinar epithelial cells have granular basophilic cytoplasm with nuclei toward the base. The submandibular is a mixed gland and contains mucinous acini topped by serous crescents. The mucinous cells have pale vacuolated cytoplasm. The sublingual gland is also mixed, though predominantly mucinous. The acini of the major salivary glands drain into intercalated ducts, which are lined by cuboidal epi-

thelium and surrounded by myoepithelial cells. These intercalated ducts drain into striated ducts that are lined by columnar cells and finally into excretory ducts lined by pseudostratified, columnar, epithelial cells. The minor glands are predominantly mucinous in type, draining via short ducts into the adjacent mucosal surfaces.

Cytologically, aspirates from normal parotid tissue show ducts and acini, and often entire lobular units with attached acini may be seen (Figs. 6-1 and 6-2). The ductal epithelial cells are smaller, with cytoplasm that stains orangeophilic by Papanicolaou method. When viewed *en face*, such cells have a honeycomb appearance. Acinar cells may be serous, mucinous, or oncocytic. Serous cells have vacuolated basophilic cytoplasm with purple granules and small, round, basally located nuclei. Mucinous cells have round nuclei, and their cytoplasm appears clear and may contain mucus vacuoles. Oncocytes are seen with advancing age and may be ductal or acinar in origin. They have abundant granular cytoplasm with well-defined cell borders and a small, round, regular nucleus with a distinct nucleolus. Acinar cells are often associated with myoepithelial cells, which have small spindle- to oval-shaped nuclei that are usually seen in a different plane of focus than acinar cells.

I. Ramzy and D. R. Mody: Department of Pathology, Baylor College of Medicine, and The Methodist Hospital, Houston, TX 77030.

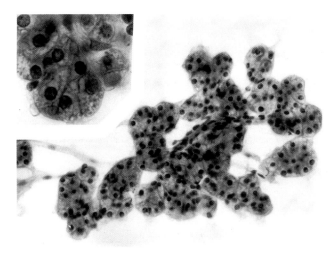

FIG. 6-1. Normal parotid gland. The acinar structures are often attached to each other. They consist of triangular cells with uniform round nuclei (*inset*). The dark cytoplasmic secretory granules usually stain purple with the Papanicolaou method and blue with Diff-Quik. (Papanicolaou stain, ×180; *inset*, ×900)

DEVELOPMENTAL AND NONNEOPLASTIC DISEASES

Cysts

Cysts account for 2% to 5% of parotid lesions. They are rare in other salivary glands. Cysts have to be distinguished from cystic salivary gland neoplasms. Benign cysts are classified histologically as lymphoepithelial, salivary duct, and dysgenic.[1]

Lymphoepithelial cysts are lined by squamous, columnar, cuboidal, or respiratory type of epithelium, and their walls contain lymphoid tissue, which can show reactive changes. The cysts are separated from the salivary gland by a zone of fibrosis, and some cysts are believed to be of branchial cleft origin. Aspiration of lymphoepithelial cysts usually results in a clear fluid that contains benign cuboidal or columnar cells, with lymphocytes (Fig. 6-3).

Salivary duct cysts usually arise on the basis of partial or complete obstruction of a large salivary duct and are lined by ductal type epithelium with rare mucus cells. Some chronic inflammation may be present in their walls. They are usually 1 to 3 cm in diameter and mostly affect patients over 40 years of age. Fine needle aspiration (FNA) of these cysts yields turbid to clear fluid that contains histiocytes, lymphocytes, few or no inflammatory cells, and some lining cells.

Other cystic lesions that can occur adjacent to salivary glands include mucoceles, mucus *escape* reactions, branchial cleft cysts, and epidermal inclusion cysts.

After the initial aspiration of any cystic lesion, it is important to palpate the area for any residual mass and reaspirate any such mass to exclude the presence of a cystic neoplasm. Pleomorphic adenomas, Warthin's tumors, mucoepidermoid carcinomas, acinic cell carcinomas, and squamous cell carcinomas can all show central cystic degeneration. If no mass is felt and reaspiration only yields normal salivary tissue, then the patient can be followed. However, if a residual mass is present, surgical management is required.[2]

Infections

Sialadenitis can be acute, subacute, chronic, or granulomatous and usually involves the parotid and submandibular glands.

Acute sialadenitis is characterized by diffuse and painful enlargement of the gland, and the overlying skin shows changes of cellulitis. Aspiration yields granulo-

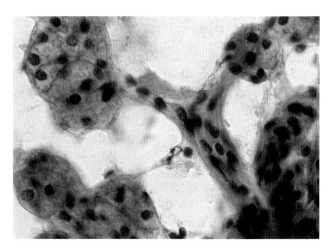

FIG. 6-2. Normal salivary gland. Finely vacuolated acinar cells arranged in tightly cohesive clusters with attached ductal elements. (Papanicolaou stain, ×360)

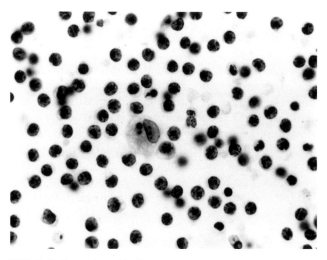

FIG. 6-3. Lymphoepithelial salivary gland cyst. The cellular aspirate consists of mature lymphocytes with scant macrophages. (Papanicolaou stain, ×900)

cytes and necrotic debris as well as some salivary acinar tissue.

Subacute and chronic sialadenitis usually present as a firm mass involving part or all of the salivary gland and can clinically mimic neoplasms. Aspiration may yield scanty material, particularly if the infection is long standing or follows radiation with fibrosis. The aspirates in such cases consist of chronic inflammatory cells intermingled with benign ductal and acinar elements with some atypia (Fig. 6-4). Although these atypical elements may be of concern, they can be distinguished from salivary gland neoplasms because their patterns are different from those described later in this chapter. The acinar units are tightly clustered, with only a few single cells, and the ductal epithelium appears as sheets of reactive and reparative cells.[3–6]

Granulomatous sialadenitis can involve the salivary glands, with tuberculosis being the most frequent infectious agent. In about 6% of cases of sarcoidosis, the salivary glands are involved, resulting in asymptomatic enlargement of the major glands as well as the intraparotid or periparotid lymph nodes.[7] Aspiration of glands involved by granulomatous sialadenitis yields benign salivary gland elements with chronic inflammation. The absence of background necrosis is an important feature. The diagnostic cells are epithelioid and multinucleated histiocytes. The epithelioid histiocytes are plump with cigar-shaped, elongated, and indented nuclei, thus giving them a reniform shape. The chromatin is vesicular with small single or multiple nucleoli. The cytoplasm is abundant, delicate, and mostly basophilic. The multinucleated histiocytes are rounded or polygonal with multiple

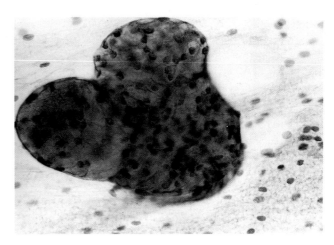

FIG. 6-5. Adenomatoid hyperplasia. The aspirate shows mucinous acinar structures and naked nuclei in a background of mucin. A rare squamous epithelial cell, derived from the overlying pseudoepitheliomatous hyperplasia, may be suggestive of a low-grade mucoepidermoid tumor. (Papanicolaou stain, ×360) (Aufdemorte TB, Ramzy I, Holt RG, et al. Focal adenomatoid hyperplasia of salivary glands: a differential diagnostic problem in fine needle aspiration biopsy. Acta Cytol 1985;29:23)

nuclei. In addition to these cells, fragments of fibrous tissue are also seen. The presence of necrosis suggests tuberculosis, whereas its absence should raise the possibility of sarcoidosis. The cytologic findings have to be taken in conjunction with clinical and other laboratory data before a diagnosis of sarcoidosis is made for the first time.

Adenomatous Hyperplasia

Adenomatous hyperplasia is an uncommon, idiopathic, usually bilateral lesion involving the minor salivary glands of the oral cavity. The lesions present as asymptomatic masses on the hard palate or retromolar trigone, covered by intact mucosa with a bluish hue. Hyperplasia can be clinically and cytologically mistaken for a salivary gland neoplasm, particularly low-grade mucoepidermoid carcinoma. The bulk of the lesion consists of a proliferation of clustered aggregates of mucinous minor salivary gland acini, some of which appear hypertrophic, but they are accompanied by normal ducts. The overlying squamous epithelium often shows pseudoepitheliomatous hyperplasia.[8,9]

Aspiration yields intact as well as ruptured acini and bare acinar nuclei, in a mucinous background that is continuous with the contents of the acini. A layer of spindle-shaped myoepithelial cells surrounds some of the intact acini. Occasional ductal epithelial cells are also seen (Fig. 6-5). Aspiration of the pseudoepitheliomatous areas yields squamous epithelium, and hence the confusion with low-grade mucoepidermoid carcinoma (Table 6-1).[10,11]

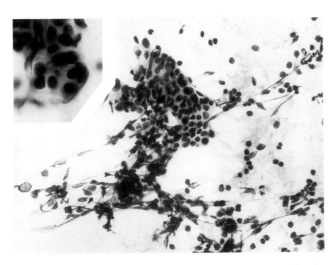

FIG. 6-4. Chronic sialadenitis. The aspirate shows a background of lymphocytes and plasma cells. The sheet of epithelial cells in the center reveals some nuclear hyperchromasia and pleomorphism, which is more evident at higher magnification (*inset*). Aspirates from benign lymphoepithelial lesions show similar cytologic features. (Papanicolaou stain, ×180; *inset*, ×900)

TABLE 6-1. *Mucoepidermoid tumor and adenomatoid hyperplasia*

Mucoepidermoid tumor	Adenomatoid hyperplasia
Predominantly in parotid, unilateral	Minor glands in palate, usually bilateral
Not uncommon	Extremely rare
Few neoplastic squamous cells	Squamous cells absent or rare
Slight cellular pleomorphism	Uniform cells
Duct cells absent or exceptional	Few duct cells
Few acinar formations	Abundant acini

(Ramzy I. Clinical cytopathology and aspiration biopsy. Norwalk, CT, Appleton & Lange, 1990:306)

Benign Lymphoepithelial Lesions

A benign lymphoepithelial lesion presents as an asymptomatic or mildly painful swelling of the parotid or submaxillary gland. It can also involve minor salivary glands and is more common in women in their fifth and sixth decades. It is usually associated with Sjögren's syndrome, although cystic variants of these lesions have been seen in patients with AIDS.[12] The glands show varying degrees of replacement of the acinar tissue by lymphocytic infiltrate and epimyoepithelial islands. Reactive germinal centers can be seen as well as plasma cells.[1]

Aspiration of benign lymphoepithelial lesions reveals a polymorphous population of small and large reactive lymphocytes, tingible body macrophages, and plasma cells (Fig. 6-6). The epimyoepithelial islands can be scarce and widely interspersed and may require careful searching. They are characterized by small clusters or loose groups of mildly atypical ductal cells surrounded by lymphohistiocytic elements. If the epithelial elements are not found and the lymphoid population appears monotonous, malignant lymphoma should be considered in the differential, and appropriate material should be sent

for marker and gene rearrangement studies if indicated (see Chap. 4). Reactive intraparotid lymph nodes should also be considered in the differential diagnosis because they also lack the epimyoepithelial islands (Table 6-2).[5,13]

Heterotopic and Accessory Salivary Glands

Heterotopic salivary gland tissue can be found in paraparotid lymph nodes, soft tissues of the neck, in the middle ear, and in other locations less frequently.[1] Accessory parotid tissue refers to salivary tissue that is separated from the main body of the gland but drains into the Stensen duct. Tumors and inflammatory processes can involve these tissues, with low-grade mucoepidermoid carcinoma being the most common malignant neoplasm.[1]

Necrotizing Sialometaplasia

Necrotizing sialometaplasia is a benign, necrotizing, self-healing inflammatory condition commonly affecting the minor salivary glands of the palate. The lesions present as deep crater-like ulcers or as 1- to 3-cm nodular swellings that ulcerate and spontaneously heal over a few weeks. Histologically, the lesion is characterized by lobular necrosis with preservation of the lobular architecture and squamous metaplasia of the residual ductal and acinar units. These lesions may be misinterpreted as squamous cell carcinoma or low-grade mucoepidermoid carcinoma in cytologic and histologic samples. Careful attention to the clinical picture, preservation of the lobular architecture, lack of mucin cysts and bland nature of the metaplastic cells, and the presence of a mixed inflammatory background should help in diagnosing these lesions correctly.[1]

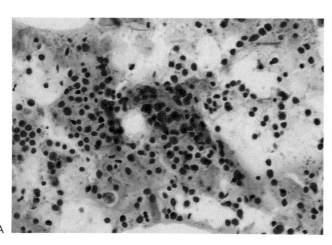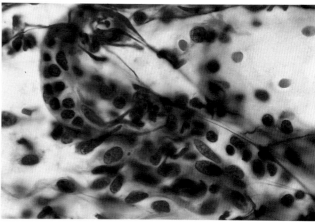

A   B

FIG. 6-6. Lymphoepithelial lesion. Ductal and acinar structures infiltrated by lymphocytes. (**A**, Papanicolaou stain, ×180; **B**, Papanicolaou stain, ×900)

TABLE 6-2. *Lymphoid infiltrates in salivary gland swellings*

Lymphoepithelial lesion	Warthin's tumor	Malignant lymphoma
GLANDS		
Salivary and lacrimal	Almost limited to parotid	Any
SITE		
Multiple, bilateral	Unilateral	Unilateral or bilateral
MASS		
Solid or partially cystic	Cystic, mucoid	Solid
LYMPHOCYTES		
Polymorphous	Polymorphous	Monomorphous
HISTIOCYTES		
Reactive	Reactive	Atypical
ONCOCYTES		
Few	Abundant	None

(Ramzy I. Clinical cytopathology & aspiration biopsy. Norwalk, CT, Appleton & Lange, 1990:304)

BENIGN NEOPLASMS

Pleomorphic Adenoma (Mixed Salivary Tumor)

Pleomorphic adenoma is the most common tumor of major and minor salivary glands, and accounts for 60% to 70% of all parotid, 40% to 60% of submandibular, and 40% to 70% of minor salivary gland neoplasms (Table 6-3). The incidence is slightly higher among women, and all ages are affected, but the most common age of onset is between 30 to 50 years. Clinically, pleomorphic adenomas present as painless, slowly growing masses. In the parotid, they usually involve the superficial lobe (90%).

TABLE 6-3. *Prevalence of 13,749 salivary gland neoplasms from the AFIP files*

Benign (%)		Malignant (%)	
Pleomorphic		Mucoepidermoid	12.4
adenoma	50.0	Acinic cell	6.4
Warthin's	5.3	Adenocarcinoma NOS	6.2
Adenoma NOS	2.4	Adenoid cystic	
Oncocytoma	1.5	carcinoma	4.4
Cystadenoma	1.4	Malignant mixed	
Basal cell adenoma	1.2	tumor	2.4
Canalicular		Squamous cell	
adenoma	0.9	carcinoma	1.6
Other benign	0.5	Other malignant	
		tumors	3.4
TOTALS	63.2		36.8

AFIP, Armed Forces Institute of Pathology; NOS, not otherwise specified.

(Adapted from Ellis GL, Auclair PL, Gnepp DR. Surgical pathology of the salivary glands. Philadelphia, WB Saunders, 1991:144)

Although the tumor appears well circumscribed, tiny microscopic foci extend along the septa and account for the high recurrence rates if the entire lobe is not removed. The adenomas consist of epithelial and stromal elements. The epithelial elements are ductal in origin and can show oxyphilic or squamous metaplasia. The stromal elements are thought to be myoepithelial in origin and can be loose myxomatous, chondroid, or spindle shaped.

FNA yields gelatinous material with abundant cellularity. The diagnostic feature is the intermingling of the epithelial and stromal elements (Fig. 6-7). On Diff-Quik staining, the background stains a bright magenta because of the hyaluronic acid-rich stroma (Fig. 6-8A). The epithelial cells have small, blue, regular nuclei and appear

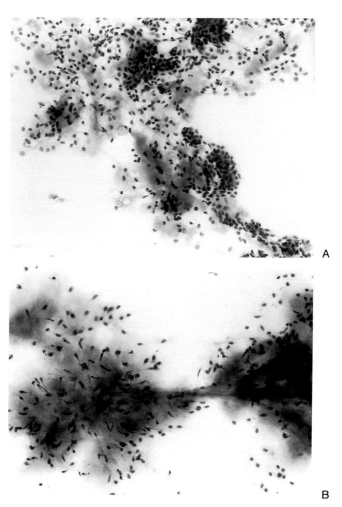

FIG. 6-7. Pleomorphic adenoma. **(A)** At low power, nests of dark epithelial cells are seen among stromal background. Observe the abundance of isolated bare nuclei. The epithelial nuclei may show slight pleomorphism, but the smear lacks the necrosis or marked nuclear atypia that characterizes carcinoma ex-pleomorphic adenoma. (Papanicolaou stain, ×180) **(B)** The myxochondroid stroma stains dark purple and is more evident in this air-dried, Diff-Quik–stained smear. Note the melting of the epithelial clusters into the surrounding stroma. (Diff-Quik stain, ×360)

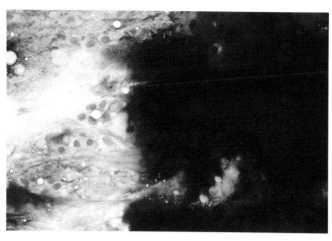
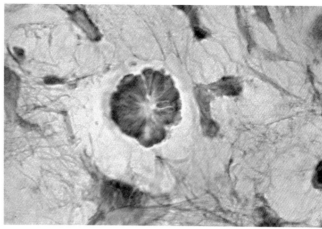

A   B

FIG. 6-8. Pleomorphic adenoma. **(A)** Brilliant magenta coloration of the background and stromal elements are diagnostic of pleomorphic adenoma. (Diff-Quik stain, ×360) **(B)** A tyrosine crystal in an aspirate from a pleomorphic adenoma. Observe the daisy petal configuration. (Papanicolaou stain, ×900)

singly, in sheets, or as arborizing ductal structures. On Papanicolaou staining, the background is less dramatic. The epithelial elements merge into the spindle-cell stroma, which is gray-green, fibrillar, and may appear chondroid. Rarely, tyrosine or collagen-rich crystalloids may be seen on aspirates (see Fig. 6-8**B**). These crystals usually have been associated with benign salivary gland tumors, particularly pleomorphic adenomas. Hyaline cell adenoma is a variant of pleomorphic adenoma in which the predominant cell is a plasmacytoid epithelial cell with hyaline eosinophilic cytoplasm.[14] The epithelial elements of pleomorphic adenomas can show squamous or oxyphilic metaplasia as well as some atypia. Such moderate atypia does not warrant the diagnosis of malignancy; carcinoma ex pleomorphic adenoma is rare, and is usually in the form of undifferentiated carcinoma, which is easy to recognize as malignant. The main differential diagnostic consideration for pleomorphic adenomas is an adenoid cystic carcinoma, and such differentiation may be difficult if only Papanicolaou-stained material is available for evaluation (Table 6-4). Rarely, adenoid cystic carcinomas arise in a pleomorphic adenoma.[15]

Monomorphic Adenoma

The term *monomorphic adenoma* is confusing because it is used to include several types of benign epithe-

lial neoplasms. Among the lesions included are basal cell adenomas and canalicular adenomas, with the former accounting for 1.8% of benign epithelial salivary gland neoplasms encountered in the Armed Forces Institute of Pathology (AFIP) files.[1] Compared with pleomorphic adenomas, monomorphic adenomas tend to occur in an older patient population, with a mean age of 57 years. About 73% occur in the parotid gland, and the neoplasms are clinically indistinguishable from pleomorphic adenomas. Histology reveals a well-encapsulated mass in which the basaloid cells are arranged in solid, trabecular, tubular, and membranous patterns. The basaloid cells have two morphologic forms: (1) small cells with dark nuclei and scant cytoplasm and (2) large cells with ovoid pale nuclei and amphophilic to eosinophilic cytoplasm. The small cells are peripherally located, and, unlike pleomorphic adenomas, there is a sharp demarcation between the epithelial elements and the surrounding connective tissue.

FNA yields cellular smears containing cohesive groups of epithelial cells, some of which may have three-dimensional and branching arrangements (Fig. 6-9). The individual cells have small regular nuclei with scant cytoplasm. Although a small amount of homogeneous metachromatic stroma may be seen at the edge of some cell groups on Diff-Quik–stained slides, the abundant fibrillar stroma and other stromal elements, seen in pleomorphic adenoma, are lacking.[16,17] The trabecular

TABLE 6-4. *Differential diagnosis of common salivary gland neoplasms*

Pleomorphic adenoma	Adenoid cystic carcinoma	Mucoepidermoid carcinoma
Epithelial cells single or loosely cohesive, medium-sized	Epithelium in three-dimensional groups of small basaloid cells with bland nuclei	Syncytial arrangement of mucinous, intermediate, and epidermoid cells
Fibrillary or myxoid stromal cells	Stromal cells not prominent	Stromal cells not prominent
Myxoid background stains magenta with DQ	Clean background, homogenous globules	Mucinous background stains pink with DQ

DQ, Diff-Quik or other Romanowsky stain.

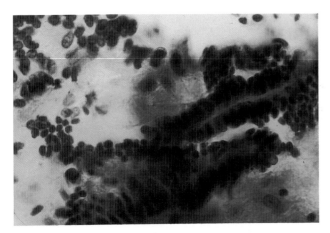

Fig 6-9. Monomorphic adenoma (canalicular type). Cellular aspirate with "ductal" formations. Note the uniformity of the neoplastic cells. (Papanicolaou stain, ×360. Courtesy of Yener S. Erozan, M.D., The Johns Hopkins University, Baltimore)

variants may be confused with adenoid cystic carcinomas because they may contain hyaline globules, but these stain blue with Romanowsky stains, unlike the pink basement membrane–type material of adenoid cystic carcinomas.[18]

Warthin's Tumor

Warthin's tumor is a benign neoplasm that is also referred to as *papillary cystadenoma lymphomatosum* or *adenolymphoma*. In 95% of cases, the tumor occurs in the lower portion of the parotid gland, accounting for 5% of all parotid neoplasms. The male/female ratio has been reported between 5:1 and 1.4:1.[1] The tumor usually presents as a soft, 3- to 5-cm, painless mass with ill-defined borders and is bilateral in 5% to 14% of cases. Cut section reveals a well-encapsulated, tan to red mass with single or multiple cystic spaces that contain clear, mucoid, or hemorrhagic fluid. Histology reveals columnar epithelial cells with underlying cuboidal cells arranged in two cell layers. Both columnar and cuboidal cells contain regular, darkly stained nuclei with small nucleoli. The epithelial elements can undergo oncocytic, squamous, or mucinous metaplasia. Under the epithelial layer are lymphocytes that can form follicles.

FNA yields a small amount of clear to turbid liquid that contains granular and amorphous debris with oncocytic epithelial cells. These cells form monolayered sheets with well-defined cytoplasmic borders. The abundant granular cytoplasm is green on Papanicolaou-stained slides and pink on Diff-Quik–stained slides. The nuclei are small and regular with small, regular nucleoli. Lymphocytes are scattered in the background (Fig. 6-10). Occasional papillary fragments with columnar cells and underlying lymphocytes are seen. Metaplastic squamous cells with atypia may be seen in some cases.

A helpful feature in Romanowsky stained smears is the presence of mast cells superimposed on sheets of oncocytes. Mast cells, which have round, dark nuclei and prominent, dark red, cytoplasmic granules, are present in 80% of Warthin's tumors. They are helpful in differentiating Warthin's tumors from branchial cysts, squamous cell carcinoma, and mucoepidermoid carcinoma.[19] The diagnostic accuracy by FNA for Warthin's tumor has been reported in the 61% to 81% range[20,21] and increases with the experience of the performer and interpreter of the smears. Occasionally, FNA results in infarction of the tumor.[22]

Oncocytoma

Oncocytoma is a relatively uncommon neoplasm accounting for 1% of all salivary gland neoplasms and 2.3% of all benign epithelial salivary gland tumors. Patients are usually in the sixth to the ninth decades.[1] Clinically, it presents as a painless, firm, lobulated mass usually in the superficial lobe of the parotid gland and may have central cystic areas. The neoplasm consists of oncocytes arranged in sheets, nests, or trabeculae. The cells are large polyhedral or round with well-defined, abundant, granular eosinophilic cytoplasm. The cytoplasmic granularity is attributed to the densely packed mitochondria. The nuclei may show some degree of atypia.

FNA yields a cellular specimen that consists of uniform large cells. These can be arranged in sheets or acini or as a syncytium of nuclei in a background of ruptured

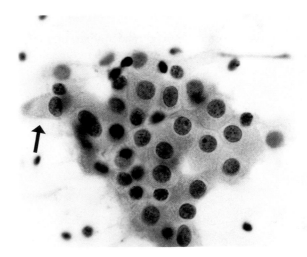

FIG. 6-10. Warthin's tumor. A sheet of oncocytes, with well-defined cell borders, is seen with a few lymphocytes in the background. The nuclei of the oncocytic cells are round or slightly oval and often display prominent nucleoli and slight pleomorphism. The abundant granular cytoplasm stains pink with Diff-Quik and is eosinophilic or cyanophilic with the Papanicolaou smear method. Most cells are polygonal, but the arrow points to a more columnar oncocytic cell. (Papanicolaou stain, ×900)

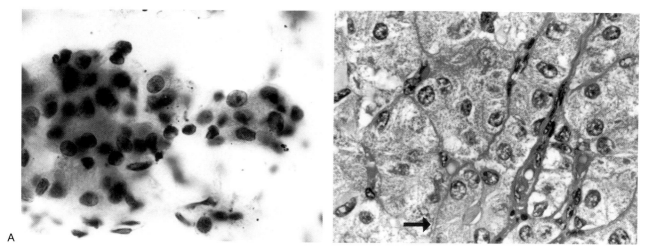

A   B

FIG. 6-11. Oncocytoma. **(A)** The neoplastic cells have abundant granular cytoplasm. The nuclei show a moderate degree of pleomorphism and some prominent nucleoli. (Papanicolaou stain, ×900) **(B)** The histologic section shows an attempt by the neoplastic cells (*arrow*) to form acini. (Hematoxylin–eosin stain, ×900)

cytoplasm (Fig. 6-11). The abundant granular cytoplasm stains green with the Papanicolaou stain and gray with the Diff-Quik stain. The nuclei are round with prominent nucleoli (Fig. 6-12). The background lacks the lymphocytes or debris seen in Warthin's tumor. Other differential diagnostic considerations include pleomorphic adenoma and mucoepidermoid carcinoma. Lack of chondroid matrix, mucinous, tubular, and squamous cells, after adequate sampling, should help overcome the difficulty in diagnosis.

Other Benign Neoplasms

Clear cell adenomas, sebaceous adenomas, and other benign epithelial neoplasms may develop in the salivary glands, but they are extremely rare and will not be con-

sidered further. Mesenchymal neoplasms such as lipomas, atypical lipomas, hemangiomas, and schwannomas can also involve the salivary glands (Fig. 6-13). Their cytologic features are similar to those encountered in soft tissues.

MALIGNANT NEOPLASMS

Adenoid Cystic Carcinoma

Adenoid cystic carcinoma is a slowly growing malignant tumor that affects both the major and minor salivary glands. It is the fourth most common malignant salivary gland tumor, accounting for 11.8% in the AFIP

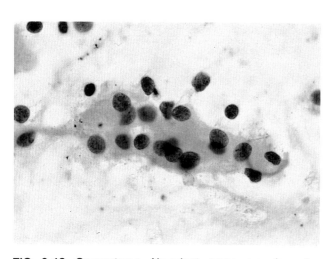

FIG. 6-12. Oncocytoma. Abundant, green, granular cytoplasm with eccentrically placed nuclei and easily identifiable nucleoli. (Papanicolaou stain, ×900)

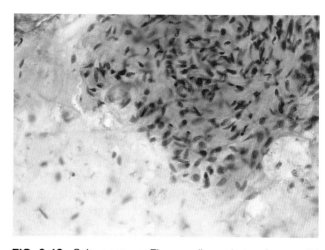

FIG. 6-13. Schwannoma. Fine needle aspirate of a parotid mass revealing a haphazard collection of cells with wavy nuclei in a somewhat myxoid background. (Papanicolaou stain, ×360. Courtesy of Mary R. Schwartz, M.D., Baylor College of Medicine, Houston)

series.[1] It affects adults in the fifth, sixth, and seventh decades of life, presenting as a slowly growing, firm, solid mass that may be painful. The long-term prognosis in incompletely excised tumors is poor; perineural involvement, local recurrence as well as pulmonary, nodal, and osseous metastases are common. The tumor cells have scant cytoplasm and may be arranged in one or more of three patterns: cribriform, tubular, and solid. In the cribriform pattern, the cells form nests of variable sizes, with round or oval central spaces. These spaces contain amorphous eosinophilic basement membrane material that is positive on periodic acid–Schiff (PAS) stain and diastase resistant. The tubular pattern has tubular and ductal structures containing similar basement membrane material. The solid type, regarded as the poorly differentiated variety, shows solid nests of cells without the spaces or basement membrane material. Unlike solid basal cell adenomas, it has foci of necrosis, greater nuclear pleomorphism, and nucleoli.

FNA yields solid particles and some liquid. The tumor cells are usually arranged in tight clusters and cell balls, which, on focusing, reveal globules within their central spaces that correspond to the basement membrane material (Fig. 6-14). The globules are diagnostic, and they stain pink with Diff-Quik or other Romanowsky stains (Fig. 6-15A) and clear or pale green on Papanicolaou stain (see Fig. 6-15B). Some of the cells form ductal or tubular structures, whereas others are arranged singly. The nuclear chromatin is pale and finely granular with a smooth nuclear membrane, and nucleoli are inconspicuous or small (see Fig. 6-15B). The cytoplasm is scant and the nuclear/cytoplasmic ratio is high. Aspirates from the solid variants lack the diagnostic globules and may be mistaken for basal cell adenoma. Careful search for even a single diagnostic cluster is warranted. In addition, the nuclei in the solid variants are larger, have coarser chromatin, and show nucleoli, features that are not seen in basal cell adenomas.[2,13,15] Layfield[18] described blue mucus balls in trabecular adenomas compared with the pink ones in adenoid cystic carcinoma when stained with Romanowsky stain. Other small cell malignant neoplasms and pleomorphic adenomas can cause diagnostic problems. The latter can have areas mimicking adenoid cystic carcinomas, and, in such instances, a diagnosis of

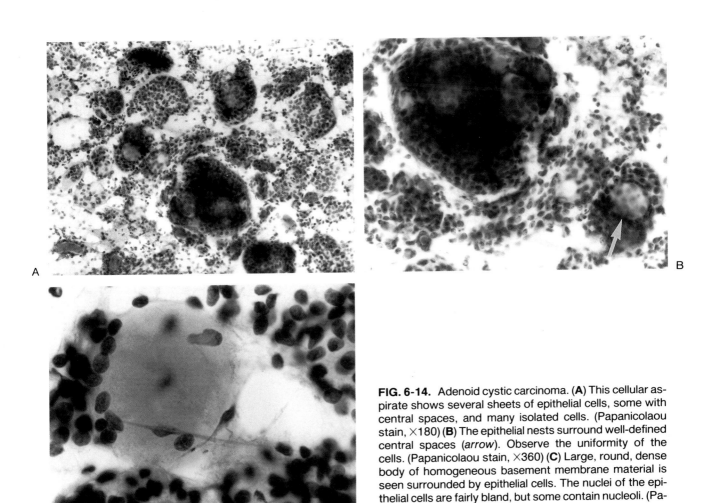

FIG. 6-14. Adenoid cystic carcinoma. **(A)** This cellular aspirate shows several sheets of epithelial cells, some with central spaces, and many isolated cells. (Papanicolaou stain, ×180) **(B)** The epithelial nests surround well-defined central spaces (*arrow*). Observe the uniformity of the cells. (Papanicolaou stain, ×360) **(C)** Large, round, dense body of homogeneous basement membrane material is seen surrounded by epithelial cells. The nuclei of the epithelial cells are fairly bland, but some contain nucleoli. (Papanicolaou stain, ×900)

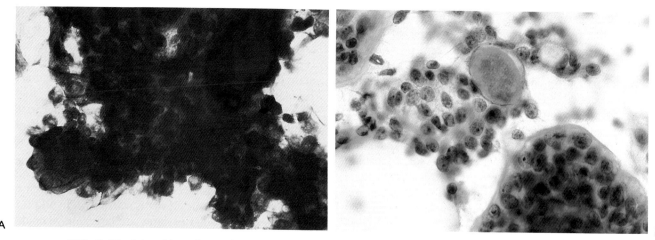

FIG. 6-15. Adenoid cystic carcinoma. **(A)** Metachromatically stained globules surrounded by uniform, basaloid cells. (Diff-Quik stain, ×360) **(B)** Three-dimensional and flat sheets of small basaloid cells with occasional nucleoli. Notice the green, basement membrane–like material. (Papanicolaou stain, ×900)

pleomorphic adenoma should be suggested with a note that open biopsy or frozen section should be obtained before any radical surgical treatment.

Mucoepidermoid Carcinoma

Mucoepidermoid carcinoma is the second most frequent salivary gland neoplasm and the most common malignant one. It affects patients from the second through the eighth decades of life.[1] About 54% occur in the major salivary glands, where they present as asymptomatic masses. Most of the remaining cases involve intraoral minor glands and are incidentally discovered during dental examinations. These neoplasms can be of low, intermediate, or high grade of malignancy, with the low-grade carcinomas having an excellent prognosis if completely excised. Several cell types are encountered in mucoepidermoid carcinomas: mucinous, epidermoid,

intermediate, columnar, and clear. Low-grade tumors show prominent cystic spaces lined by mucinous cells and abundant extracellular mucin. Intermediate and epidermoid cells are present in smaller numbers. Intermediate-grade tumors show fewer cystic spaces with a predominance of the smaller intermediate cells. High-grade tumors are solid neoplasms and show proliferation of atypical epidermoid and intermediate cells, whereas mucinous cells are difficult to find.

FNA of low-grade mucoepidermoid carcinomas yields mucinous or blood-tinged fluid. The smears reveal a mixture of intermediate and mucin-secreting cells, with only a few squamous cells; the background often is mucinous (Fig. 6-16). The glandular cells are columnar or oval, with pale-staining cytoplasm containing mucin. The nuclei are eccentrically located and have fine chromatin and small nucleoli. The intermediate cells are small, have scant eosinophilic cytoplasm and small

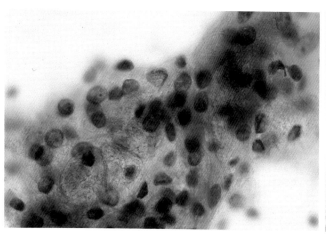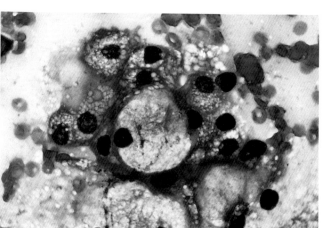

FIG. 6-16. Mucoepidermoid carcinoma. **(A)** Papanicolaou stain demonstrating the intermediate and the mucin-producing cells. (Papanicolaou stain, ×900) **(B)** The latter are often better appreciated on the Diff-Quik–stained material. (Diff-Quik stain, ×900)

round nuclei (Fig. 6-17). Metaplastic squamous cells may also be seen. Aspiration of high-grade tumors does not yield any liquid. However, the smears are cellular and cytologically resemble a squamous cell carcinoma. Mucinous and intermediate cells are difficult to find, and in the absence of these, a definitive diagnosis of muco-epidermoid carcinoma cannot be made.[23,24]

Low-grade mucoepidermoid carcinomas must be distinguished from necrotizing sialometaplasia and chronic sialadenitis, both of which usually yield scant cellularity and have an inflammatory background. Mucoceles are acellular or contain histiocytes and inflammatory cells, and the cystic lesions disappear after aspiration, leaving no residual masses behind. Differentiation from adenomatoid hyperplasia has been previously discussed. High-grade carcinomas may be cytologically indistinguishable from a squamous cell carcinoma metastasizing to the salivary gland from an occult head and neck primary. Although mucin stains may be of some help, metastatic carcinoma should be clinically ruled out because the management of both lesions is different.

Acinic Cell Adenocarcinoma

Acinic cell adenocarcinoma is a malignant neoplasm that is mostly encountered in the parotid gland (83%) and less frequently in submandibular and other salivary glands. The tumors are thought to arise from cells at the intercalated ducts. The mean age at presentation is 44 years, and they result in slow growing solid or cystic masses that are usually well circumscribed and may be multinodular. Most neoplasms consist of acinar cells, but other components may be encountered, such as in-

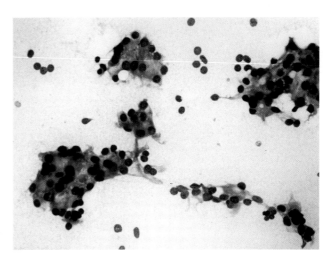

FIG. 6-18. Acinic cell carcinoma. The neoplastic cells are attempting to form acini. Although acinic cell tumors are considered malignant, the cells usually have fairly bland nuclei. Because of the fragile nature of acinic cells, many rupture during the preparation of smears, leaving an abundance of bare nuclei. Observe the absence of duct cells and the limited tendency of the acini to cluster, unlike aspirates from normal glands illustrated in Figure 6-1. (Papanicolaou stain, ×360)

tercalated duct-like, vacuolated, or clear cells. The cells are arranged in solid, microcystic, papillary cystic, or follicular patterns. The cuboidal intercalated duct-like cells are smaller than acinar cells, and they surround small lumina. Although their nuclei are similar to those of acinar cells, they have a higher nuclear/cytoplasmic ratio. The vacuolated cells are the size of acinar cells, but their cytoplasm is distended by multiple or single vacuoles that do not stain for mucin, lipids, or other substances.

FNA may yield a small amount of fluid, in addition to fragments from the solid areas, producing abundantly cellular smear. The large acinar cells are arranged in sheets or ill-defined loose acinar structures, but in many cases they appear as isolated cells. They have abundant foamy or gray cytoplasm on Diff-Quik staining and small and regular dark eccentric nuclei with nucleoli. The cytoplasm contains PAS-positive, diastase-resistant granules.[25] Additionally, the background shows many bare acinar nuclei and lymphocytes (Figs. 6-18 and 6-19). Although the cells are similar to those of a normal salivary gland, fat cells and ductal epithelial cells are not usually encountered in acinic cell neoplasms. In poorly differentiated acinic cell carcinomas, nuclear pleomorphism with large nucleoli are encountered. Acinic cell carcinomas are usually associated with a lymphoid infiltrate, which may be mistaken for a lymph node, and in such cases the possibility of Warthin's tumor should also be considered.[26] However, the oncocytic cells in Warthin's tumor are arranged in sheets and not in acinar formations. The PAS reaction is also helpful because acinic cells are PAS-positive and diastase resistant. Mast cells are absent in acinic cell carcinomas.

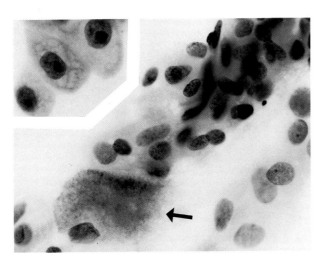

FIG. 6-17. Mucoepidermoid tumor. Aspirate from this intermediate-grade neoplasm shows a mucinous cell (*arrow*) with granular precipitated mucin in the cytoplasm, mixed with benign-looking squamous cells. Inset shows three intermediate cells with multiple mucinous vacuoles in their cytoplasm. (Papanicolaou stain, ×900; *inset*, ×900)

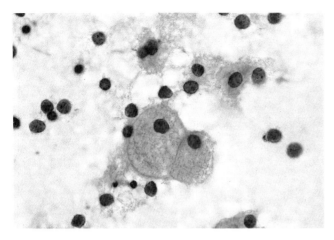

FIG. 6-19. Acinic cell carcinoma. Loose groups of finely vacuolated acinar-like cells with bare nuclei in the background that resemble those seen in the intact cells. This is due to the rupture of the fragile cytoplasm. Contrast this picture with that of normal salivary gland as seen in Figure 6-2. (Papanicolaou stain, ×900)

Adenocarcinoma Not Otherwise Specified

The third most common group of malignant tumors of the salivary glands encompasses adenocarcinomas that cannot be further classified. Such neoplasms ac-

count for 17.4% of all malignant epithelial salivary gland tumors and 6.4% of all salivary gland tumors.[1,27]

About 50% involve the parotid, 10% involve the submaxillary, and the remainder involve the palatal and oral minor salivary gland tissue. The diagnosis is that of exclusion because the tumors do not fit the pattern of any of the usual neoplasms. They can have tubular, trabecular, solid, or other growth patterns. The fine needle aspirate shows features of usual adenocarcinomas (Fig. 6-20). High-grade tumors may be mistaken for undifferentiated carcinomas, whereas low-grade tumors may be misdiagnosed as benign.

Squamous Cell Carcinoma

Primary squamous cell carcinomas account for 4.4% of all malignant epithelial salivary gland tumors. Seventy-five percent involve the parotid, with the mean age of the patient being 60 years.[1,27] Histologically and cytologically they resemble squamous cell carcinomas from other sites (Fig. 6-21). Differential diagnostic considerations include ductal squamous metaplasia, necrotizing sialometaplasia, high-grade mucoepidermoid carcinoma, and metastatic squamous cell carcinoma.

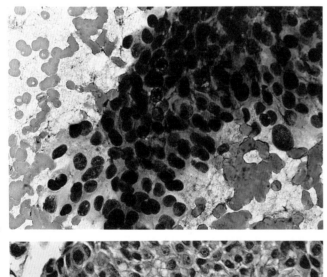

A

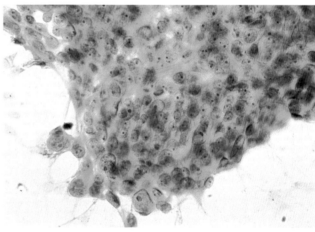

B

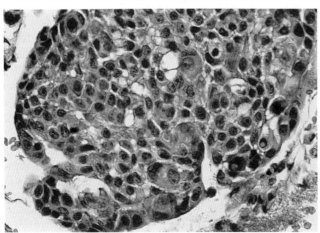

C

FIG. 6-20. Adenocarcinoma. This poorly differentiated adenocarcinoma arising from the submandibular gland does not have any cytologic features of specific types of salivary gland carcinomas (ie, adenoid cystic, mucoepidermoid, or acinic cell carcinomas). (**A,** Diff-Quik stain, ×360; **B,** Papanicolaou stain, ×360; **C,** Cell block, hematoxylin–eosin stain, ×360. Courtesy of Yener S. Erozan, M.D., The Johns Hopkins University, Baltimore)

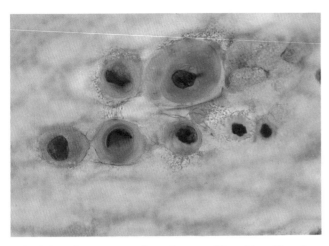

FIG. 6-21. Squamous cell carcinoma of the skin with extension into the salivary gland. Observe the extracellular mucin in the background, which can be seen occasionally in such skin lesions. Abundant extracellular mucin was also seen on review of the original resection. (Papanicolaou stain, ×900)

Undifferentiated Carcinoma

Undifferentiated carcinoma is a heterogeneous group of neoplasms that includes small cell undifferentiated carcinoma, large cell undifferentiated carcinoma, and lymphoepithelial carcinoma. Their exact incidence is difficult to determine, but in the AFIP series they account for 0.4% of salivary gland tumors.[1] They resemble their counterparts in other organs, but clinical distinction of primary versus metastatic undifferentiated carcinomas is essential because primary small cell carcinomas of the salivary gland have a better prognosis compared with their counterparts in the lung or larynx.[28,29]

Lymphomas

There has been a steady increase in the number of primary salivary gland lymphomas. They constitute 11.1% of all primary parotid malignancies in the AFIP series, with non-Hodgkin's lymphomas constituting over 97% of cases.[1,30,31] Most lymphomas arise de novo, with peak age in the seventh decade. Only a small percentage arise on the basis of preexisting lymphoepithelial lesions or Sjögren's syndrome. In patients with Sjögren's syndrome, the risk of developing lymphoma is about 40 times higher than in the control population.[31] About 75% of lymphomas occur in the parotid gland, and 60% fall into the low-grade category on the Working Formulation Group. Monocytoid B-cell lymphomas arise from mucosal associated lymphoid tissue in the minor salivary glands.[32–34] FNA yields a monomorphic population of lymphocytes, and the principles of cytologic diagnosis are similar to those used for lymph nodes (see Chap. 4).[35,36] Immunocytochemical or flow cytometric studies are essential for confirming the monoclonality of the

cells, and gene rearrangement studies may be required in some difficult cases.

Other Malignant Tumors

Some less common neoplasms may involve the salivary glands. These include clear cell carcinomas, sebaceous carcinomas, polymorphous low-grade adenocarcinomas, and others. Isolated case reports are listed in the references, and a detailed description is beyond the scope of this chapter.[37–42] Carcinoma ex pleomorphic adenoma rarely poses diagnostic difficulties.[43] Metastatic malignancies can also involve the salivary glands, the most common site being intraparotid lymph nodes. Squamous cell carcinoma and melanoma are the most common malignancies, although breast cancer, renal cell carcinoma, and others have also been reported.[44,45] If the primary source is unknown, immunocytochemistry and clinical correlation are required.[46]

CONCLUSIONS

Aspiration biopsy results in accurate diagnosis in more than 90% of pleomorphic adenomas and 60% of Warthin's tumors, the most common tumors of salivary glands. Malignant tumors form about 25% of neoplasms of the salivary glands, and about half of these are interpreted as malignant without difficulty. Proper classification, however, can be difficult and may require resection or open biopsy.

Aspiration provides several advantages to the clinician faced with a swelling of the salivary gland area. It can determine if the swelling is of salivary gland origin, if it is a tumor, and if it is benign or malignant. It also helps in planning for resection, radiotherapy, or chemotherapy, such as in case of lymphomas or anaplastic carcinoma. The surgeon can also plan to sacrifice the sensory great auricular nerve if the lesion proves to be malignant preoperatively.

Some argue that aspiration biopsy is not helpful because 75% of cases are pleomorphic adenomas. Diagnosis of lesions other than pleomorphic adenomas, however, provides information that influences management. These situations include lymph nodes with reactive hyperplasia, hyperplasia in HIV-positive patients where minimal intervention is needed, and in lymphomas and metastatic carcinomas, which require radiotherapy or radical surgery. Cysts can be diagnosed and also treated during a single visit. Aspiration also allows the search for primary sources in case of metastatic disease such as melanoma, and it gives the clinician the opportunity for proper preoperative preparation of certain tumors such as paragangliomas. Aspiration can also establish the diagnosis in poor surgical candidates, in whom resection of benign lesions such as Warthin's may not be necessary.

The tendency of pleomorphic adenomas to recur locally also raises the possibility of recurrence along the needle track. However, large series by Swedish authors have shown this to be extremely rare with fine needles. Following aspiration, the skin track can also be marked by injecting ink and excised with the tumor. The difficulty in detecting malignant transformation in pleomorphic tumors and in determining the need to sacrifice the facial nerve at the time of surgery is not unique to FNA; frozen sections do not fare better because the detection of a small focus is dependent on the extent of sampling.

Mucoepidermoid tumors can be the source of false-positive and false-negative results, and special care should be exercised in evaluating these lesions. The cell monotony of some adenoid cystic and acinic cell carcinomas can also be deceptive. The sensitivity and specificity of the technique, however, can be greatly enhanced by multiple sampling, particularly of residual tissues after aspirating a cyst.

We find staining by both Diff-Quik and Papanicolaou methods to be complementary and essential in the evaluation and correct interpretation of salivary gland lesions. Immunocytochemistry is not particularly helpful in distinguishing among the different primary salivary gland neoplasms. It does play a role, however, in the diagnosis of lymphomas and metastatic disease. Silver-staining nucleolar organizer region (AgNOR) counts have been reported in salivary gland cytology, but their usefulness in the day-to-day practice of salivary needle aspiration biopsies remains to be determined.[47]

REFERENCES

1. Ellis GL, Auclair PL, Gnepp DR. Surgical pathology of the salivary glands. Philadelphia, WB Saunders, 1991.
2. Ramzy IR. Clinical cytopathology & Aspiration Biopsy. Norwalk, CT, Appleton & Lange, 1990.
3. Kline TS, Merriam JM, Shapshay SM. Aspiration cytology of the salivary gland. Am J Clin Pathol 1981;76:263.
4. Mavec P, Eneroth CM, Franzen S, et al. Aspiration biopsy of salivary gland tumours. I. Correlation of cytologic reports from 652 aspiration biopsies with clinical and histologic findings. Acta Otolaryngol (Stockh) 1964;58:471.
5. Qizilbash AH, Sianos J, Young JEM, et al. Fine needle aspiration biopsy cytology of major salivary glands. Acta Cytol 1985;29:503.
6. Webb AJ. Cytologic diagnosis of salivary gland lesions in adult and pediatric surgical patients. Acta Cytol 1973;17:51.
7. Werning J. Infectious and systemic diseases. In: Ellis GL, Auclair PL, Gnepp DR. Surgical pathology of the salivary glands. Philadelphia, WB Saunders, 1991:51.
8. Arafat A, Brannon RB, Ellis GL. Adenomatoid hyperplasia of mucous salivary glands. Oral Surg 1981;52:51.
9. Devildos LR, Langlios CC. Minor salivary gland lesions presenting clinically as tumor. Oral Surg 1976;41:657.
10. Aufdemorte TB, Ramzy I, Holt RG, et al. Focal adenomatoid hyperplasia of salivary glands: a differential diagnostic problem in fine needle aspiration biopsy. Acta Cytol 1985;29:23.
11. Giansanti JS, Baker GO, Waldron CA. Intraoral mucinous minor salivary gland lesions presenting clinically as tumors. Oral Surg 1971;32:918.
12. Tao LC, Tullane PJ. HIV infection associated lymphoepithelial lesions of the parotid gland: aspiration biopsy cytology, histology and pathogenesis. Diagn Cytopathol 1991;7:158.
13. Geisinger KR, Weidner MD. Aspiration cytology of salivary glands. Semin Diagn Pathol 1986;3:219.
14. Schultenover SJ, McDonald EC, Ramzy I. Hyaline cell pleomorphic adenoma: diagnosis by fine needle aspiration biopsy. Acta Cytol 1984;28:593.
15. Geisinger KR, Reynolds GD, Vance RP, et al. Adenoid cystic carcinoma arising in a pleomorphic adenoma of the parotid gland: an aspiration cytology and ultrastructural study. Acta Cytol 1985;29:522.
16. Hruban RH, Erozan YS, Zinreich JS, et al. Fine needle aspiration of monomorphic adenomas. Am J Clin Pathol 1988;90:46.
17. Stanley MW, Horwitz CA, Henry MJ, et al. Basal cell adenoma of the salivary gland: a benign adenoma that cytologically mimics adenoid cystic carcinoma. Diagn Cytopathol 1988;4:342.
18. Layfield LJ. Fine needle aspiration cytology of a trabecular adenoma of the parotid gland. Acta Cytol 1985;29:999.
19. Bottles K, Lowhagen T, Miller TR. Mast cells in the aspiration cytology differential diagnosis of adenolymphoma. Acta Cytol 1985;29:513.
20. Kline TS, Merriman JM, Shapsay SM, et al. Aspiration biopsy cytology of the salivary gland. Am J Clin Pathol 1981;76:263.
21. Eneroth CM, Zajicek L. Aspiration biopsy of salivary gland tumors. II. Morphologic studies on smears and histologic sections from oncocytic tumors. Acta Cytol 1965;9:355.
22. Kern SB. Necrosis of a Warthin's tumor following fine needle aspiration. Acta Cytol 1988;32:207.
23. Linsk JA, Franzen S. Clinical aspiration cytology, ed 2. Philadelphia, JB Lippincott, 1989:103.
24. Zajicek J, Eneroth CM, Jakobsson P. Aspiration biopsy of salivary gland tumors. VI. Morphologic studies on smears and histologic sections from mucoepidermoid carcinomas. Acta Cytol 1976;20:35.
25. O'Dwyer P, Farrar WB, James AG, et al. Needle aspiration biopsy of salivary gland tumors and its value. Cancer 1986;57:544.
26. Abrams AM, Cornyn J, Scofield HH, et al. Acinic cell adenocarcinoma of major salivary glands: a clinicopathologic study of 77 cases. Cancer 1965;18:1145.
27. Eveson JW, Cawson RA. Salivary gland tumours: a review of 2410 cases with particular reference to histologic types, sites, age and sex distribution. J Pathol 1985;146:51.
28. Koss LC, Spiro S, Hajdu S. Small cell carcinoma of minor salivary gland origin. Cancer 1972;30:737.
29. Kraemer BB, Mackay B, Batsakis JG. Small cell carcinomas of the parotid gland: a clinicopathologic study of three cases. Cancer 1983;52:2115.
30. Gleeson MJ, Bennett MH, Cawson RA. Lymphomas of salivary glands. Cancer 1986;58:699.
31. Schmid U, Helbron D, Lennert K. Primary malignant lymphomas localized in salivary glands. Histopathology 1982;6:673.
32. Isaacson PG, Spencer J. Malignant lymphoma of mucosa associated lymphoid tissue. Histopathology 1987;11:445.
33. Hyjek E, Smith WJ, Isaacson PG. Primary B cell lymphoma of salivary glands and its relationship to myoepithelial sialadenitis. Hum Pathol 1988:19:766.
34. Sheibani K, Burke JS, Swartz WG, et al. Monocytoid B cell lymphoma: clinicopathologic study of 21 cases of a unique type of low grade lymphoma. Cancer 1988;62:1531.
35. Sneige N, Dekmezian R, El Naggar A, et al. Cytomorphologic, immunocytochemical, and nucleic acid flow cytometric study of 50 lymph nodes by fine needle aspiration: comparison with results obtained by subsequent excisional biopsy. Cancer 1991;67:1003.
36. Sneige N, Dekmezian R, Katz R, et al. Morphologic and immunocytochemical evaluation of 220 fine needle aspirates of malignant lymphoma and lymphoid hyperplasia. Acta Cytol 1990;34:311.
37. Rivka G, Strauss M, Zohar Y. Salivary duct carcinoma of the parotid gland: cytologic and histopathologic study. Acta Cytol 1985;29:454.
38. Batsakis JG: Clear cell tumors of salivary glands. Ann Otol Rhinol Laryngol 1980;89:196.
39. Gnepp DR. Sebaceous neoplasms of salivary gland origin. Pathol Annu 1983;18:71.
40. Hood IC, Qizilbach AH, Salama SS. Needle aspiration cytology of sebaceous carcinoma. Acta Cytol 1984;28:305.

41. Frierson HF, Covell JL, Mills SE. Fine needle aspiration cytology of terminal duct carcinoma of minor salivary gland. Diagn Cytopathol 1987;3:159.

42. Regezi JA, Zarbo RJ, Stewart JC, et al. Polymorphous low grade adenocarcinoma of minor salivary gland: a comparative histologic and immunohistochemical study. J Oral Surg Oral Med Pathol 1991;71:469.

43. Pitman MB. Mucoepidermoid carcinoma ex pleomorphic adenoma of the parotid gland. Acta Cytol 1995;39:604.

44. Conley J, Arena S. Parotid gland as a focus of metastasis. Arch Surg 1963;87:757.

45. Yarington CT. Metastatic malignant disease to the parotid gland. Laryngoscope 1981;91:517.

46. Domagala W, Lasota J, Wolska H, et al. Diagnosis of metastatic renal cell and thyroid carcinomas by intermediate filament typing and cytology of tumor cells in fine needle aspirates. Acta Cytol 1988;32:415.

47. Cardillo MR. Ag-NOR technique in fine needle aspiration cytology of salivary gland masses. Acta Cytol 1992;36:147.

Fine Needle Aspiration of Subcutaneous Organs and Masses,
edited by Yener S. Erozan and Thomas A. Bonfiglio.
Lippincott–Raven Publishers, Philadelphia, © 1996.

CHAPTER 7

Fine Needle Aspiration of Other Subcutaneous Masses and Cystic Lesions

Dina R. Mody and Ibrahim Ramzy

Subcutaneous and soft tissue lesions are fairly common and easily accessible to sampling by fine needle aspiration (FNA). Aspiration of these masses is a simple, reliable, and cost-effective means of establishing the diagnosis. Most subcutaneous masses are visible or palpable and hence can be directly aspirated using a 25-gauge needle. Deeper masses require visualization by radiographic or other techniques to guide the aspiration. In our laboratory, air-dried and alcohol-fixed smears are prepared and stained with the Diff-Quik and Papanicolaou techniques, respectively. Cell blocks and tissue fragments, when available, are processed as paraffin blocks and are most helpful for immunocytochemical staining.

A wide variety of nonneoplastic and neoplastic subcutaneous and soft tissue lesions can be aspirated. The first part of this chapter discusses inflammatory and other nonneoplastic lesions; the second part discusses benign and malignant primary neoplasms as well as metastatic tumors.

NONNEOPLASTIC LESIONS

Inflammatory Conditions

Inflammatory lesions comprise abscesses and foreign-body and granulomatous reactions. It is important to

D. R. Mody and I. Ramzy: Department of Pathology, Baylor College of Medicine, and The Methodist Hospital, Houston, TX 77030.

recognize these various lesions at the time of FNA so that appropriate microbiologic cultures can be obtained.

Abscesses

Abscesses can be due to infection by a variety of microorganisms, but in some cases they may not be of infectious etiology. Some sterile abscesses are caused by injections and represent an exuberant foreign-body reaction to the active compound injected or its diluent.[1] In the latter situation, the foreign material is seen within histiocytes or free within necrotic fat.

Granulomatous Inflammation

When granulomas result in subcutaneous nodules, they are easy targets for FNA. The smears are characterized by an inflammatory background with or without necrosis. Epithelioid and multinucleated histiocytes are the diagnostic cells. Epithelioid cells are plump, with vesicular, elongated nuclei with indentations in their longitudinal axis, resulting in a reniform shape. Single to multiple small, regular nucleoli may be seen. The cytoplasm is abundant, delicate, and usually pale basophilic with ill-defined cell borders. The multinucleated histiocytes are larger than epithelioid cells, and fibrous tissue fragments are interspersed through these aggregates (Fig.

7-1). Appropriate special stains can be used to reveal any organisms that may be responsible for the granulomas. Leprosy,[2] leishmaniasis,[3] granuloma inguinale,[4] coccidioidomycosis, and tuberculosis,[5] are among the infections that can be diagnosed. Sarcoidosis is another granulomatous inflammatory condition that can be diagnosed in the appropriate clinical scenario.[6]

Other Nonneoplastic Conditions

A wide variety of masses that are not inflammatory or neoplastic in nature may be encountered in aspirates. These include keloids, scars and fibrosis, fat necrosis, radiation-induced changes, epithelial inclusion cysts, branchial cleft cysts, and ganglion cysts. The group also includes nodular and proliferative fasciitis and myositis, as well as some less common lesions such as endometriosis, supernumerary breasts, and amyloidosis.

Keloids, Scars, and Fibrosis

Keloids and scars that develop at sites of previous cancer resection are occasionally aspirated if recurrence is suspected. They yield scant cytologic material consisting of spindly fibroblastic cells and collagen fibers. If such lesions happen to be in the field of radiation, cytologic atypia of the stromal cells may be observed. Such changes are similar to those described previously. The pathologist should ascertain that the nodule has been adequately sampled before concluding that it is a scar because some carcinomas may induce a dense desmoplastic response.

Epithelial Inclusion Cysts

Epithelial inclusion cysts yield benign squamous epithelial cells that are predominantly anucleated. If rup-

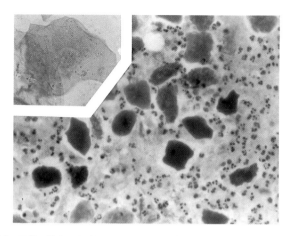

FIG. 7-2. Epithelial inclusion cyst. Note the anucleated and superficial squamous cells and debris. Rupture of the cysts can induce intense inflammatory and foreign-body reaction. Inset demonstrates an anucleated squame. (Papanicolaou stain, ×180; *inset*, ×900)

tured, the keratinous contents often incite a most exuberant foreign-body and inflammatory reaction (Fig. 7-2).

Branchial Cleft Cysts

Branchial cleft cysts usually occur in the neck and are lined by squamous or columnar epithelium. Aspiration reveals benign squamous or columnar epithelial cells with some lymphocytes and other chronic inflammatory cells (Fig. 7-3). If branchial or epidermal inclusion cysts are located in the field of radiation of a previous squamous cell carcinoma, they may be associated with prominent epithelial atypia and should not be mistaken for recurrent tumor.[7]

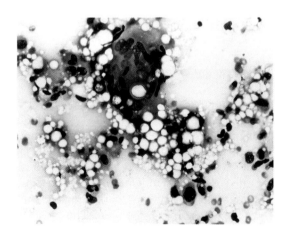

FIG. 7-1. Postinjection granuloma. Refractile material, appearing as vacuoles, is seen within histiocytes and foreign-body giant cells. The foreign material in this case was silicone. (Papanicolaou stain, ×180)

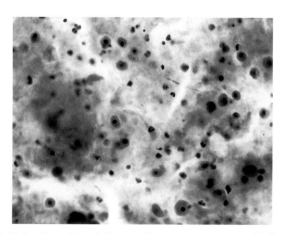

FIG. 7-3. Branchial cleft cyst. Note the necrotic and inflammatory debris admixed with squamous cells, columnar cells, and lymphocytes. (Papanicolaou stain, ×180)

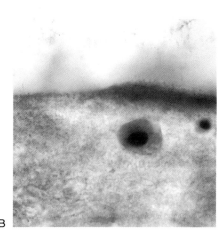
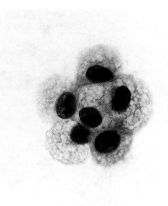

A,B

FIG. 7-4. Ganglion cyst. **(A)** The hypocellular specimen consists of myxomatous background and a rare, benign, histiocyte-like cell. **(B)** Several vacuolated cells with uniform nuclei. (**A** and **B**, Papanicolaou stain, ×900)

Ganglion Cysts

Ganglions occur most frequently in the dorsum of hands and wrist. Although the usual treatment is surgical excision under local or general anesthesia, FNA of these is both diagnostic and therapeutic and yields colorless to pale yellow gelatinous fluid. Cytologically, the smears are fairly monotonous with abundant mucoid material, few collagen fibers, few red blood cells, and a variable number of histiocytes arranged singly or in clusters (Fig. 7-4).[8,9]

Fat Necrosis

Fat necrosis is characterized by the presence of necrotic adipocytes with a varying admixture of fibrocytes and histiocytes, some of which may be multinucleated. The adipocytes are in various stages of disintegration with cloudy cytoplasm, often appearing as "ghost" fat cells. The histiocytes have finely vacuolated cytoplasm and occasionally have enlarged hyperchromatic nuclei. Attention to the smooth nuclear outline and the abundant vacuolated cytoplasm is helpful in distinguishing these from malignant cells, particularly liposarcomas and renal cell carcinomas (Fig. 7-5).

Radiation-Induced Changes

Cytologic changes may be seen anywhere from within days after radiotherapy to years after radiation for malignant disease. Palpable masses may be aspirated to rule out recurrence of the malignancy. Apart from the presence or absence of viable or necrotic tumor, three patterns may be encountered in the nonneoplastic tissue caught in the field of radiation: (1) epithelial atypia, (2) fat necrosis, and (3) scant cellularity without atypia or fat necrosis. The epithelial atypia is characterized by cytomegaly, anisocytosis, anisonucleosis, occasionally prominent nucleoli but a normal nuclear/cytoplasmic ratio. Nuclear and cytoplasmic vacuolation may also be seen.

Fat necrosis is seen occasionally with radiation, whereas in many post-radiation cases, the smears are poorly cellular, with rare benign stromal cells and no atypia.[10]

Nodular Fasciitis

A benign, rapidly growing lesion, nodular fasciitis is often mistaken clinically, histologically, and cytologically for a sarcoma. In young adults, it usually occurs on the upper extremity, chest, and back; in children, however, it is seen in the head and neck. The cell yield on cytology depends on the age of the lesion. Most aspirates are cellular, consisting of plump spindle and stellate cells having large, oval, often eccentric nuclei with mild hyperchromasia and one to two nucleoli. The cells are single or in loose clusters and have well-defined cytoplasm. Increased mitotic activity but without atypical mitosis is seen. The mucoid background surrounding the interwoven bundles of fibroblasts is best seen as blue to reddish purple material by Diff-Quik stain. Scattered lymphocytes and macrophages, some with hemosiderin pigment, may also be encountered.[11] Older lesions show hyaline fibrosis, tissue shrinkage, and a central fluid-filled space and they yield scant cellular material.

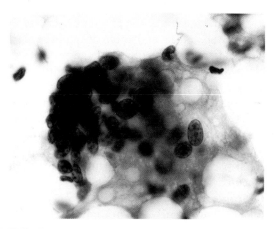

FIG. 7-5. Fat necrosis. Giant cell with ingested fat. (Papanicolaou stain, ×360)

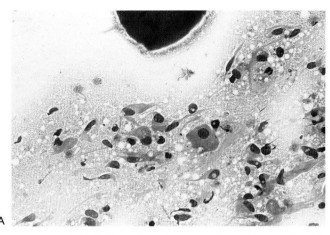
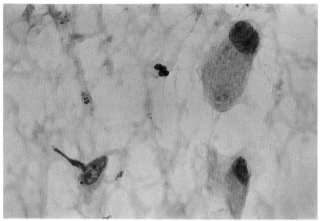

A   B

FIG. 7-6. Proliferative myositis. (A) Plump fibroblasts and larger ganglion-like cells in a granular background. Note the degenerating skeletal muscle fiber at the 12-o'clock location. (Hematoxylin–eosin stain, ×180) (B) Plump fibroblasts and ganglion-like cells with eccentric nuclei and nucleoli in a granular to myxoid background with a rare inflammatory cell. (Papanicolaou stain, ×900)

Other Nonneoplastic Lesions

Proliferative fasciitis and myositis are related self-limiting, benign, but rapidly growing lesions in subcutaneous fat and muscle of adults. The mean age of the patient with proliferative myositis (sixth decade) is older than that of patients with nodular fascitis. The proliferating fibroblasts intermingle with plump basophilic giant cells resembling ganglion cells or rhabdomyoblasts. Fine needle aspirates reveal these cells in a myxoid background (Fig. 7-6). The large ganglion-like cells may be mistaken for the giant cells of malignant fibrous histiocytoma (MFH). However, MFH cells are more irregular in form, nuclei, and chromatin pattern. An open biopsy is often necessary to determine the nature of these lesions, and thorough knowledge of the clinical, histopathologic, and cytopathologic features should lead to the correct diagnosis, thus avoiding surgical resection.

Fibromatosis comprises a broad group of fibrous tissue proliferations that, in their biologic behavior, are intermediate between benign fibrous lesions and fibrosarcoma. They may occur in the palmar or plantar fascia, abdominal wall, neck, and other locations. They are characterized histologically by a benign proliferation of fibroblasts with interstitial collagen and infiltrative properties. FNA yields scanty material that on smears shows rare fibroblasts, acellular collagen, naked nuclei, and damaged cells.[12] Some cases of fibromatosis, such as desmoid tumors, yield more cellular material but with similar cytologic features. Occasionally, it is difficult to distinguish between fibromatosis and low-grade spindle cell sarcoma on cytologic grounds alone.

Other miscellaneous lesions may be encountered in the subcutaneous tissues. Laparotomy scars may be involved by endometriosis. In such cases, needle aspirates yield a cellular smear with a background of neutrophils and histiocytes with interspersed syncytial clusters of loosely cohesive endometrial cells, forming groups of 2 to 15 cells per cluster, or they may be seen singly. Mucinous metaplasia may be encountered in endometriotic foci. Three-dimensional epithelial clusters, characteristic of endometrial cells in exfoliative specimens, are not seen in aspirates.[13,14] Supernumerary breasts may be encountered along the "milk lines," and they tend to enlarge during pregnancy (Fig. 7-7). FNA reveals benign clusters of acinar cells that may show prominent nuclei and nucleoli if associated with pregnancy.[15]

FNA biopsy of abdominal fat pad has also been reported to be a good screening procedure in patients at risk for amyloidosis. Cell blocks can be prepared for electron microscopy, whereas immunofluorescence can be performed on smears. Positive staining with an alkaline Congo red and apple green birefringence is diagnostic

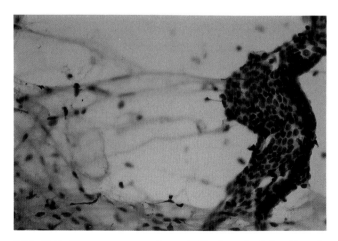

FIG. 7-7. Supernumerary breast. Benign ductal cells admixed with adipose tissue in an aspirate from a nodule along the milk line. (Papanicolaou stain, ×360)

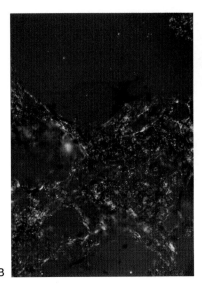 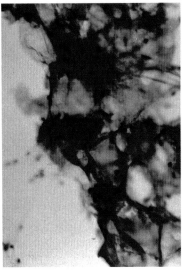

A,B

FIG. 7-8. Amyloid. **(A)** Apple green birefringence characteristic of amyloid. Note the amyloid fibrils are short and numerous and follow the contours of the adipocyte nuclei. **(B)** Abdominal fat pad aspirate demonstrating congophilia on alkaline Congo red staining. **(A** and **B,** Congo red stain [**A** under polarized light], ×360)

when performed on air-dried smears (Fig. 7-8). The true amyloid fibrils are short and follow the contours of the adipocytes, unlike collagen bundles, which are thicker and bandlike and do not follow cell contours.[16]

Tumoral Calcinosis

Tumoral calcinosis is a benign condition and can be associated with hyperparathyroidism or renal disease. Occasionally, no predisposing condition exists; patients in this group tend to be younger, and the presence of such masses has a familial basis. The masses appear along the extensor surfaces of extremities and tendon sheaths. The radiographic appearance is usually diagnostic. However, the lesions may be large and mimic a bone neoplasm. In these instances, aspiration is helpful, yielding calcified debris with rare histiocytes and foreign-body giant cells (Fig. 7-9).

Bursitis

Aspiration of bursae yields thick fluid and fronds of papillary synovial hyperplasia in patients with bursitis. The synovial cells are histiocytic in origin with a normal nuclear/cytoplasmic ratio, bland chromatin, and occasional nucleoli (Fig. 7-10).

NEOPLASMS

Fibrohistiocytic Tumors

Benign Fibrous Histiocytoma

Benign fibrous histiocytomas (eg, dermatofibromas, xanthofibromas) occur in the dermis and superficial subcutis, particularly in the extremities. The amount of ma-

FIG. 7-9. Tumoral calcinosis. Aspirate of elbow mass showing calcium and rare histiocytes. (Papanicolaou stain, ×900)

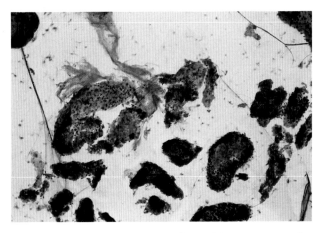

FIG. 7-10. Bursitis. Aspiration of shoulder mass revealing three-dimensional papillary fronds of synovial hyperplasia. (Papanicolaou stain, ×90)

terial obtained at FNA depends upon the age of the lesion, with fibrosis being a feature of older lesions. Short fibroblastic cells arranged in whorled clusters along with some benign single cells of similar type are seen (Fig. 7-11). The nuclei are oval with evenly distributed fine chromatin and small nucleoli. Histiocytic cells and Touton giant cells contain hemosiderin and fat. Touton giant cells have a wreath of monomorphous oval nuclei without hyperchromasia. Dermatofibromas are distinguished from low-grade MFHs by the lack of nuclear pleomorphism and mitotic activity.

Dermatofibrosarcoma Protuberans

Dermatofibrosarcoma protuberans is a neoplasm that presents as a multinodular mass on the trunk of middle-aged men. It involves the dermis and subcutaneous fat. It can be histologically and cytologically similar to dermatofibromas, but it has a tendency to recur locally if inadequately excised. FNA yields a moderately cellular specimen with cells arranged in a storiform pattern. The predominant cell type is spindle cells with rare interspersed larger polylobate cells (Fig. 7-12).

Malignant Fibrous Histiocytoma

The most common soft tissue sarcoma of adult life, MFH has a wide range of histologic appearances, including pleomorphic, myxoid, giant cell, inflammatory, and angiomatoid subtypes.[17] The last three variants are rarely encountered.

Pleomorphic MFH is the most common subtype, usually occurring during the sixth to seventh decade in the skeletal muscle of extremities or retroperitoneum. It is a high-grade sarcoma consisting of spindle and histiocyte-

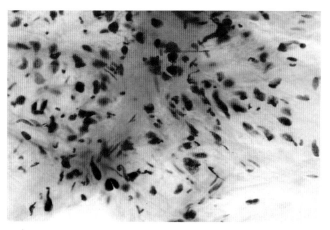

FIG. 7-12. Dermatofibrosarcoma protuberans. Needle aspirate of back mass with moderate cellularity consisting of spindle cells in a storiform arrangement and scattered larger cells with multilobate nuclei. (Papanicolaou stain, ×360)

like cells. The mitotic rate is high, and necrosis is prominent. FNA yields abundant material containing both elements. The atypical fibroblasts have large, hyperchromatic nuclei, intranuclear "holes," and one or more prominent nucleoli. They may be arranged in a cartwheel fashion. The other cell component consists of large atypical pleomorphic, histiocyte-like cells (Fig. 7-13). These are mononucleated, binucleated, or multinucleated; they are often bizarre and show ingested cell debris and lipids. Their presence helps to differentiate MFH from other pleomorphic high-grade sarcomas. Immunohistochemistry shows α_1-antitrypsin, α_1-antichymotrypsin, lysozyme, and muramidase positivity.

Myxoid MFH is a variety in which at least half of the tumor has a myxoid pattern. This variety has a better prognosis than the pleomorphic type. Cytology reveals a myxoid background in which spindle cells as well as gi-

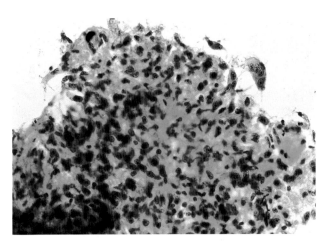

FIG. 7-11. Benign fibrous histiocytoma. Cellular aspirate from a young lesion with fibroblasts, histiocytes, and giant cells. (Papanicolaou stain, ×180. Courtesy of Yener S. Erozan, M.D., The Johns Hopkins University, Baltimore)

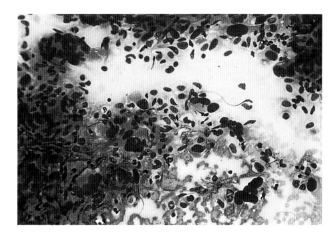

FIG. 7-13. Pleomorphic malignant fibrous histiocytoma. Cellular aspirate with atypical fibroblasts, large pleomorphic histiocyte-like cells, and multinucleated giant cells. (Diff-Quik stain, ×180. Courtesy of Yener S. Erozan, M.D., The Johns Hopkins University, Baltimore)

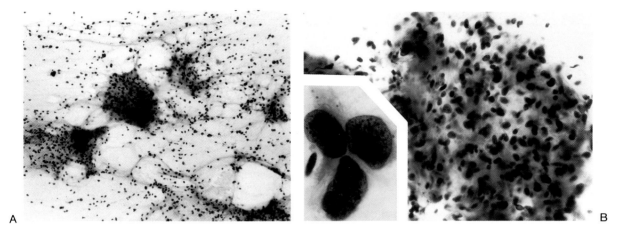

FIG. 7-14. Malignant fibrous histiocytoma. (A) The specimen is cellular, with a myxomatous background in which groups and sheets of spindle cells are identified. (B) Some cells are arranged in a storiform pattern. Large pleomorphic multinucleated cells (*inset*) are also seen. (Papanicolaou stain; **A,** ×90; **B,** ×180; *inset,* ×900)

ant cells show features similar to those of pleomorphic MFH. The cellularity of the tumor, lack of delicate vascular pattern, and absence of lipoblasts help to differentiate this type from myxoid liposarcoma, myxoma, and other tumors with myxomatous degeneration (Fig. 7-14).

Myxoid Tumors

True myxomas are rare. Most myxoid tumors encountered represent myxomatous change or a variant of other neoplasms such as MFHs, liposarcomas, neurofibrosarcomas, chondrosarcomas, chordomas, and nodular fasciitis. Sampling of different areas of myxoid lesions is critical for correct identification of their nature.

Myxomas are benign tumors that occur most frequently in the large muscles of the thigh and shoulder. They are round to oval, seemingly well-circumscribed tumors with a glistening gray-white gelatinous appearance. Fine needle aspirates yield colorless, mucoid, stringy, viscous material with scant cellularity. The background stains bluish violet by Diff-Quik stain and green-blue by Papanicolaou stain. The cells have small ovoid or fusiform dark nuclei, with scant cytoplasm that may have long cytoplasmic processes (Fig. 7-15). Occasional triangular or stellate cells as well as multivacuolated macrophages with intracytoplasmic oil red O–positive material are seen. Unlike lipoblasts, the vacuoles appear as small droplets and do not indent the nucleus. Small muscle fragments with proliferating sarcolemmal nuclei mimicking multinucleated giant cells were seen in seven out of ten cases described by Åkerman and Rydholm.[18] The main differential diagnostic considerations are listed in Table 7-1.

Lipomatous Tumors

Lipomas and liposarcomas are some of the most common soft tissue tumors. These neoplasms are characterized by accumulation of variable amounts of fat in the cytoplasm. As a result, several varieties of lipomatous neoplasms are encountered.

Lipoma

Lipomas present as slowly growing masses, often in subcutaneous tissue, skeletal muscle, bone, or retroperitoneum. They are usually encapsulated, although in deeper tissues like skeletal muscle they may have infil-

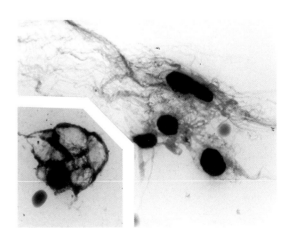

FIG. 7-15. Intramuscular myxoma. Hypocellular specimen in which rare spindle cells as well as cells with abundant vacuolated cytoplasm (*inset*) are seen. The vacuoles, unlike those of lipoblasts, are small and do not indent the nucleus. (Air-dried, Diff-Quik stain, ×900; *inset,* ×900)

TABLE 7-1. *Differential diagnosis of myxomatous neoplasms*

Tumor	Location	Cellularity/ background	Cell type	Other
Ganglion cyst	Hands, wrist, extremities	Scant cells, myxoid background	Vacuolated histiocyte-like cells	—
Myxoma	Intramuscular	Extremely low cellularity, myxoid background	Spindle or polygonal with or without vacuoles	Oil red O +ve vacuoles that do not indent nuclei
Myxoid liposarcoma	Extremities, retroperitoneum	Highly cellular, myxoid background with arborizing vessels	Vascular network with lipocytes and lipoblasts	Oil red O +ve vacuoles that indent nuclei
Myxoid malignant fibrous histiocytoma	Extremities, retroperitoneum	Highly cellular, myxoid and necrotic	Spindle and pleomorphic, multinucleated	Lysozyme, muramidase α_1-antitrypsin +ve
Myxomatous degeneration in tumors	Depends on tumor	Depends on tumor, myxoid background	Spindle or other	Look for specific features of tumor

trative margins. Lipomas with smooth muscle and vascular elements (angiomyolipomas) commonly occur in the kidneys, whereas those with hematopoietic elements (myelolipomas) are usually found in adrenal glands and retroperitoneum. Other rare variants of lipomas include spindle cell lipoma, hibernoma, and pleomorphic lipoma.

During FNA of the common type of lipoma, there is a characteristic lack of resistance once the capsule has been penetrated, and a drop of oily liquid containing tissue fragments of mature fat cells is usually obtained. The oval nuclei of the mature adipocytes are barely visible and are present in a plane of focus different from that of the single cytoplasmic vacuole (Fig. 7-16). Without the clinical information of a well-circumscribed mass, an aspirate of normal subcutaneous tissue cannot be differentiated from that of a lipoma.

In pleomorphic lipomas, mature adipocytes and spindle cells are associated with bizarre giant cells that have multiple hyperchromatic nuclei arranged in a concentric floret fashion within a deeply eosinophilic cytoplasm. A

cytologic misdiagnosis of liposarcoma can be avoided if the clinical presentation and circumscription of the lesion are kept in mind. Lipomas can also undergo myxoid change and may be difficult to recognize as lipomas. Attention to the adipocytes in the background helps clinch the diagnosis (Fig. 7-17).

Liposarcoma

Liposarcoma is one of the most common sarcomas of adult life, with a peak incidence between the years of 40 and 60. It is found in deep tissues, particularly of the thigh and retroperitoneum. Four major histologic types are recognized: (1) well differentiated, (2) myxoid, (3) round cell, and (4) pleomorphic. The well-differentiated and myxoid types are low-grade sarcomas that tend to recur locally. The pleomorphic and round cell types are high-grade sarcomas that tend to metastasize. The atypi-

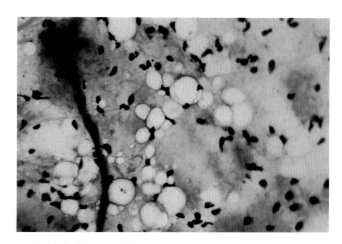

FIG. 7-17. Lipoma with myxoid change. Posterior neck mass aspirate with mature adipocytes against a myxoid background. Also interspersed are spindle cells and a rare blood vessel. (Diff-Quik stain, ×360. Courtesy of Mary Ostrowski, M.D., Baylor College of Medicine, Houston)

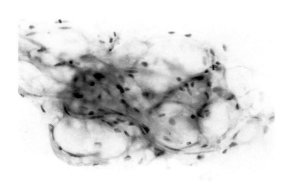

FIG. 7-16. Lipoma. Vacuolated adipocytes with nuclei pushed to the periphery of the cytoplasm. (Papanicolaou stain, ×360)

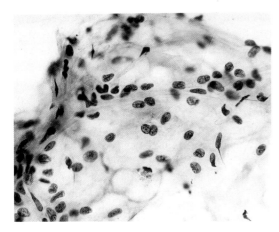

FIG. 7-18. Well-differentiated liposarcoma. Aspirate of a large retroperitoneal mass with increased cellularity and nuclear enlargement. (Papanicolaou stain, ×360)

cal multivacuolated lipoblast is the diagnostic cell. Other cellular and stromal elements are seen, depending upon the type of liposarcoma.

Well-Differentiated Liposarcoma

Well-differentiated liposarcoma exhibits a spectrum varying from lipoma-like areas to areas with nuclear pleomorphism in univacuolated adipocytes. Other areas show preadipocytes and classic lipoblasts (Fig. 7-18). Sampling several areas of the tumor to avoid misdiagnosing these as lipomas is important.

Myxoid Liposarcoma

Myxoid liposarcomas account for 40% to 50% of liposarcomas and comprise (1) proliferating lipoblasts in varying stages of differentiation, (2) a delicate plexiform capillary network, and (3) a myxoid matrix rich in hyaluronidase-sensitive mucopolysaccharides. FNA yields moderately cellular samples with a green-blue myxoid background on Papanicolaou stain and pink to magenta on Diff-Quik staining. Interspersed are tissue fragments in which a plexiform capillary network is evident, even on low magnification. The tumor cells are relatively small and uniform, with indistinct cytoplasmic borders. The nuclei are oval with evenly distributed chromatin and occasional small nucleoli. The cells are connected to capillaries by fine cytoplasmic processes (Fig. 7-19). Few diagnostic multivacuolated lipoblasts are seen, characterized by eccentric, scalloped, hyperchromatic nuclei surrounded by fat vacuoles of varying sizes, usually in intimate contact with the capillaries.[19,20] Differential diagnostic considerations include intramuscular myxoma, myxoid MFH, myxoid chondrosarcoma, and chordoma, all of which lack the classic lipoblasts and have other distinguishing features already discussed (see Table 7-1).

Round Cell Liposarcoma

Round cell liposarcoma is a poorly differentiated form of myxoid liposarcoma, characterized by a proliferation of small blue cells. The vascular component is less prominent as is the intercellular matrix and intracellular lipid formation. Mitotic activity is low, and transition to the myxoid form may be seen. FNA yields abundant cellular material with a mucoid background in which numerous tumor cells are embedded. The nuclei are round to oval and more irregular, hyperchromatic, and pleomorphic than in myxoid liposarcoma. The atypical multinucleated lipoblast rarely may be seen (Fig. 7-20).

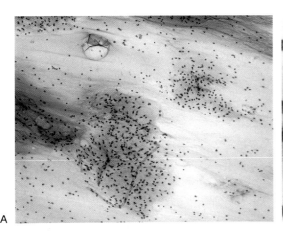 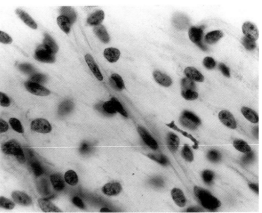

A   B

FIG. 7-19. Myxoid liposarcoma. (A) Cellular specimen with myxomatous background and arborizing vascular network, characteristic of this neoplasm. (Papanicolaou stain, ×180) (B) Perivascular clustering of preadipocytes and adipocytes, as a result of their attachment to the blood vessels. (Papanicolaou stain, ×900)

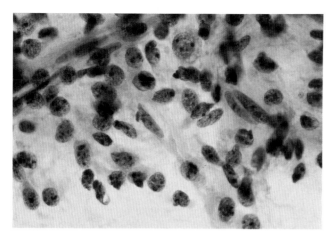

FIG. 7-20. Round cell liposarcoma. Cellular aspirate with many preadipocytes attached to a capillary. Compared with myxoid liposarcoma, the cells are larger and rounder, with prominent nucleoli. (Papanicolaou stain, ×900)

Pleomorphic Liposarcoma

Pleomorphic liposarcomas resemble any high-grade sarcoma with spindle cells, bizarre multinucleated giant cells, increased mitotic activity, and necrosis. Aspirates are usually poorly cellular, consisting mostly of necrotic debris. The viable cells show marked pleomorphism, multinucleation, and bizarre nuclei. The presence of an occasional highly atypical lipoblast helps in the diagnosis. Some lipoblasts may contain cytoplasmic hyaline globules that stain blue-gray on Diff-Quik staining. Differential diagnosis includes other high-grade sarcomas, particularly pleomorphic MFH.

Angiomatous Tumors

Angiomatous tumors include arteriovenous malformation (a nonneoplastic lesion), hemangioma, lymphangioma, hemangiopericytoma, angiosarcoma, and Kaposi's sarcoma. Aspiration of the first three lesions is not advised and yields mostly blood or lymph, with a rare spindly endothelial cell. The vascular nature of these tumors can be determined on immunocytochemistry by factor VIII and *Ulex europaeus* positivity. The presence of elements other than endothelial cells should be carefully ruled out before the diagnosis of angioma is rendered, because endothelial cells are often seen in aspirates from other masses such as liposarcomas or reactive lymph nodes.

Angiosarcoma

Angiosarcomas account for less than 1% of all soft tissue sarcomas. About one third occur in the skin and may

be associated with lymphedema. Angiosarcomas also occur in the breast and soft tissues. Cutaneous angiosarcomas are characterized by interconnecting vascular channels that split tissue planes and infiltrate. FNA of well-differentiated tumors yields scant, cytologically benign spindle cells in a bloody background. The poorly differentiated tumors are richly cellular and cytologically malignant.[21-25] Cell blocks are particularly helpful, and the endothelial nature of the cells is proved immunocytochemically by factor VIII–related antigen and *U europaeus* positivity. More recently, CD31 and CD34 are found to be helpful in the diagnosis of high-grade angiosarcomas that may mimic any carcinoma, melanoma, or sarcoma. Although CD34 is sensitive, it is not as specific. CD31, on the other hand, is highly sensitive and specific.[26] Hence, in high-grade angiosarcomas, in which testing for factor VIII and *U europaeus* is invariably negative, CD31 proves valuable. In limited aspiration samples, cell transfer followed by immunocytochemistry for CD31 has been helpful in our experience (Fig. 7-21).[27]

Kaposi's Sarcoma

A multifocal, low-grade sarcoma, Kaposi's sarcoma commonly occurs on the skin and mucosal surfaces in patients with acquired immunodeficiency syndrome (AIDS). A classic form unassociated with AIDS also occurs. Clinically, it presents as solitary or multiple reddish brown to bluish nodules that coalesce to form plaques. The cytologic picture is similar to that of angiosarcoma. The tumor cells may be spindled or plump and form slit-like spaces filled with blood. Immunohistochemically, they are positive for factor VIII–related antigen and *U europaeus*-lectin. The diagnosis of Kaposi's sarcoma on limited cytologic material should be made with caution, particularly in HIV-positive patients, because this results in an unequivocal diagnosis of AIDS.

Smooth Muscle Tumors

Smooth muscle tumors commonly occur in the uterus and gastrointestinal tract. The superficial varieties occur in the skin and subcutaneous tissue and are much less common.

Leiomyoma

Benign smooth muscle neoplasms of soft tissue are composed of interlacing bundles of spindle-shaped smooth muscle cells. FNA yields poorly cellular material consisting of solid cell clusters and occasional single cells. The nuclei are oval to elongated, with regular, smooth, nuclear outlines and finely dispersed chromatin. Differential diagnostic considerations include other spindle

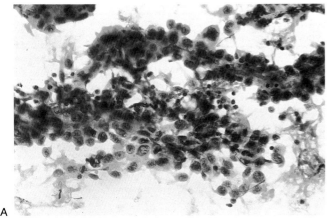

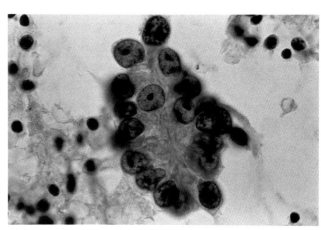

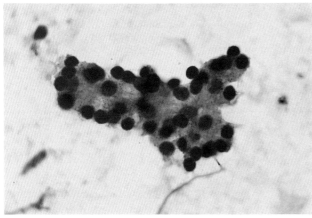

FIG. 7-21. High-grade angiosarcoma. **(A)** Cellular aspirate from an erythematous periparotid lesion. Note the malignant cells attached to vascular channels. (Papanicolaou stain, ×180) **(B)** Acinar or wreathlike arrangement of cells with large nuclei and nucleoli. Such arrangements have been described in high-grade angiosarcomas and can result in a misdiagnosis of adenocarcinoma. Notice the presence of lymphocytes in the background. (Papanicolaou stain, ×900) **(C)** Positivity of the tumor cells for CD31 is diagnostic. (Immunocytochemical stain CD31, ×360)

cell neoplasms like fibromatosis, desmoid tumor, Kaposi's sarcoma, neurofibroma, and desmoplastic melanoma.[28] If abundant material is available, a battery of immunocytochemical stains including muscle-specific actin and desmin should be performed to demonstrate the smooth muscle differentiation.

Leiomyosarcoma

Leiomyosarcomas of the skin and subcutaneous tissues account for 2% to 3% of all superficial soft tissue sarcomas. Due to their superficial location, they have a better prognosis than deeply seated leiomyosarcomas. They may be low- or high-grade sarcomas, and their cytologic features are similar to leiomyosarcomas of the female genital tract. The differential diagnosis of these tumors from other spindle cell malignancies is outlined in Table 7-2.

Skeletal Muscle Tumors

Adult rhabdomyoma is a rare benign tumor. The malignant counterpart, rhabdomyosarcoma, falls under three histologic types: (1) embryonal, (2) alveolar, and (3) pleomorphic.

Embryonal Rhabdomyosarcoma

Rhabdomyosarcoma is most commonly embryonal. It occurs mainly in children, particularly in the head and neck, retroperitoneum, and urogenital tract. It is characterized histologically by small undifferentiated cells admixed with variable numbers of more differentiated rhabdomyoblasts. Cellular areas in the tumor may alternate with less cellular and myxoid areas. Aspirates from the cellular areas yield preparations rich in small, blue, undifferentiated cells (Fig. 7-22). Identification of the larger, better differentiated rhabdomyoblasts clinches the diagnosis. These cells are large, round, with acidophilic cytoplasm, and may show cross striations or peripheral vacuoles. Elongated "strap" cells as well as stellate forms may also be seen. In the absence of the differentiated cells, immunocytochemistry, electron microscopy, or both can help in the diagnosis (Table 7-3).

Alveolar Rhabdomyosarcoma

Alveolar rhabdomyosarcoma occurs most commonly in the extremities of children and young adults. FNA yields abundant small tumor cells singly, in clusters, or around empty spaces, mimicking an alveolar pattern. In

TABLE 7-2. *Differential diagnosis of malignant spindle cell neoplasms*

Tumor	Diagnostic feature	Immunocytochemistry and other special stains	Electron microscopy
Fibrosarcoma	Diagnosis by exclusion	Vimentin	Basal lamina, RER, IF, collagen
Leiomyosarcoma	Perinuclear vacuole +/−	Vimentin, desmin, muscle-specific actin	Basal lamina, myofilaments, dense bodies
Pleomorphic malignant fibrous histiocytoma	Pleomorphic phagocytic cell	Vimentin, α_1-antitrypsin, α_1-antichymotrypsin, lysozyme, muramidase	Lysozomes, phagocytic vacuoles, attachment plaques
Neurofibrosarcoma	Neural or schwannian differentiation	Vimentin, S-100	Basal lamina, microfilaments, microtubules
Pleomorphic liposarcoma	Lipoblast	Vimentin, S-100, Oil red O	Lipoblast
Pleomorphic rhabdomyosarcoma	Rhabdomyoblast	Vimentin, sarcomeric actin, desmin, muscle-specific actin, trichrome (Z band)	Myofilaments, Z bands, sarcomeres
Angiosarcoma		Vimentin, factor VIII, *Ulex europaeus,* CD31, CD34	Weibel Palade bodies, pinocytotic vesicles, basal lamina, tight junctions
Synovial sarcoma	Gland formation helpful	Keratin, vimentin, carcinoembryonic antigen in epithelial areas	Small lumina with microvilli, cell junctions
Spindle squamous cell carcinoma	—	Keratin	Desmosomes, tonofilaments
Spindle cell melanoma	Melanin	S-100, HMB-45	Melanosomes (rare)

RER, rough endoplasmic reticulum; IF, intermediate filaments.

the absence of rhabdomyoblasts, the differential diagnostic considerations are those of a small blue cell tumor.

Pleomorphic Rhabdomyosarcoma

Pleomorphic rhabdomyosarcoma is a rare, highly malignant tumor of adults characterized by markedly pleomorphic cells of various shapes and sizes. Demonstration of cross-striations is diagnostic, as is the immunocytochemical demonstration of myoglobin or sarcomeric actin. Cytologically, it is a pleomorphic high-grade sarcoma to be distinguished from other pleomorphic sarcomas like MFH and liposarcoma.

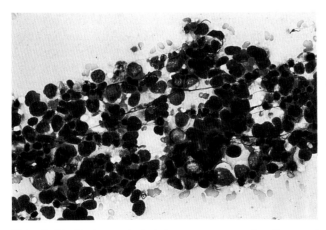

FIG. 7-22. Embryonal rhabdomyosarcoma. Small, round cells with high nuclear/cytoplasmic ratios in a necrotic background. (Diff-Quik stain, ×360. Courtesy of Yener S. Erozan, M.D., The Johns Hopkins University, Baltimore)

Tumors of Peripheral Nerves

Traumatic neuromas, benign nerve sheath tumors, and neurofibrosarcomas are the tumors of the peripheral nerves. Aspiration of these lesions characteristically elicits severe and sudden pain in the distribution of the affected nerve, often distant from the actual site of the needle.

Traumatic Neuroma

Traumatic neuromas are not true neoplasms. They result from proliferation of the axon nerve sheath complex at the site of amputation or trauma. The result is a disordered mass of axons, fibroblasts, and Schwann cells. Aspiration yields scant material comprising a few nondiagnostic spindle cells. Taking a proper history and evaluation of clinical features are usually helpful in arriving at the correct diagnosis.

Benign Nerve Sheath Tumors

Benign nerve sheath tumors include neurofibroma and schwannoma. They occur as solitary lesions in young adults but may be associated with Recklinghausen's disease, in which case there is a 25% tendency of malignant transformation. Neurofibromas are circumscribed and composed of thin, faintly eosinophilic, spindle cells lying in a collagenous matrix. Aspirates yield uniform spindle cells that are S-100 positive. Occasional nuclear palisading may be seen. Schwannomas are encapsulated, and, in addition to the spindle cells of

TABLE 7-3. *Immunocytochemistry of small blue cell tumors*

	Keratin	Vimentin	LCA	O13*	NSE	Chromagranin	Muscle-specific actin
Neuroendocrine Ca	+/−	−	−	−	+	+	−
Lymphoma	−	+/−	+	−	−	−	−
Rhabdomyosarcoma	−	+	−	−	−	−	+
Neuroblastoma	−	−	−	−	+	+	−
Ewing's sarcoma	−	+/−	−	+	+	−	−

LCA, leukocyte common antigen; NSE, neuron-specific enolase.
* Data from Weidner N, Tjoe J. Immunohistochemical profile of monoclonal antibody O13. Am J Surg Path 1994;18:486.

Antoni A component and loose Antoni B areas, they may show Verocay bodies. These bodies have polarized, elongated, vesicular nuclei and finely granular chromatin (Fig. 7-23).[29]

Neurofibrosarcoma

Malignant nerve sheath tumors may be solitary and sporadic, or they may be associated with neurofibromatosis, in which case they may be multiple. The overall organization is that of fibrosarcomas with a herringbone pattern. Densely cellular areas may alternate with hypocellular and myxomatous areas. High-grade tumors may have areas resembling MFH. Aspiration yields cellular samples in which the cells are arranged in fascicles— loosely cohesive clusters—as well as singly. The cells are mostly fusiform to plump spindle, with oval to elongated nuclei. These are hyperchromatic, with chromatin clumping and irregular nuclear outlines. Mitotic figures, necrosis, and bare nuclei are seen. Other heterotopic components such as rhabdomyoblasts (malignant triton tumor) and glandular and epithelioid elements may be seen. Immuno-

histochemistry reveals S-100 positivity in some cells (Fig. 7-24). Differential diagnostic considerations include other spindle cell sarcomas (Table 7-4).[30–32]

Tumors of Uncertain Histogenesis

Granular Cell Tumor

Granular cell tumors usually involve the tongue, skin, and subcutaneous tissue, but may affect skeletal muscle and the gastrointestinal and respiratory tracts. Aspiration yields moderate cellularity with the cells being arranged singly or in loose clusters. The individual cells are large (30 to 60 μm) and polygonal, elongated, or oval with distinct cell borders (Fig. 7-25). The cytoplasm is abundant and contains clearly visible granules that are periodic acid–Schiff (PAS)-positive and diastase resistant. The nuclei are uniform in shape and centrally or eccentrically located.[33] These tumors should be differentiated from storage diseases, rhabdomyoma, alveolar soft part sarcoma, and paraganglioma.[21,34,35] Malignant

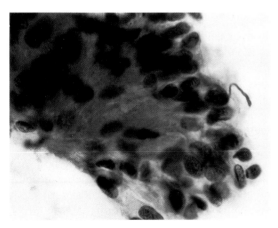

FIG. 7-23. Benign nerve sheath tumor. A three-dimensional cluster of spindle cells with palisading of nuclei, characteristic of Verocay bodies of a schwannoma. (Papanicolaou stain, ×900)

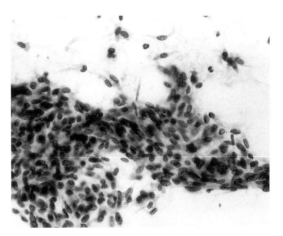

FIG. 7-24. Neurofibrosarcoma. Hypercellular specimen with hyperchromatic spindle cells arranged singly (*arrow*) and in bundles. Immunocytochemistry showed S-100 positivity. (Papanicolaou stain, ×360)

TABLE 7-4. *Immunocytochemistry of spindle cell tumors*

	Keratin	Vimentin	S-100	HMB-45	Sarcomeric actin	Desmin	Muscle-specific actin
Melanoma	−	+/−	+	+	−	−	−
Squamous carcinoma	+	+/−	−	−	−	−	−
Rhabdomyosarcoma	−	+	−	−	+	+	+
Neurofibrosarcoma	−	+	+	−	−	−	−
Leiomyosarcoma	−	+	−	−	−	+	+
Synovial sarcoma	+	+	−	−	−	−	−
Fibrosarcoma	−	+	−	−	−	−	−

granular cell tumors are uncommon and show considerable cellular pleomorphism including giant cells.

Alveolar Soft Part Sarcoma

Usually affecting the extremities or the head and neck, alveolar soft part sarcomas are rare tumors of adolescents and young adults; they have a predilection for females. The tumor is characterized by sharply defined islands of tumor cells separated by thin-walled vascular channels. FNA yields cellular smears with the cells lying singly or in aggregates with a pseudoalveolar pattern. The cells are large and round or polygonal, with abundant finely granular eosinophilic or vacuolated cytoplasm. The nuclei are vesicular with prominent, usually single, nucleoli and scant mitotic activity (Fig. 7-26A). PAS-positive, diastase-resistant crystalline material is seen in the cytoplasm (see Fig. 7-26B), and electron microscopy shows the rod-shaped crystalloid bodies.[36] Rhomboid crystals with a regular lattice pattern of 100-A periodicity may also be seen. Differential diagnosis includes metastatic renal cell carcinoma, paraganglioma, and granular cell tumor. The PAS stain is diagnostic.[37–39]

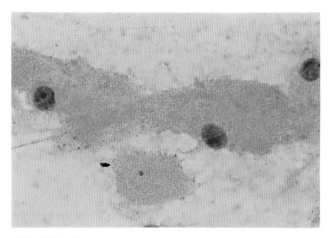

FIG. 7-25. Granular cell tumor. Aspiration of this breast lesion reveals cells with low nuclear/cytoplasmic ratios and abundant, granular, cyanophilous cytoplasm. (Papanicolaou stain, ×900)

Primary Tumors of the Skin and Appendages

The value of cytodiagnosis in dermatology has been a subject of several studies.[40,41] Basal and squamous cell carcinomas, melanomas, primary adnexal tumors, and lymphomas have been diagnosed by FNA or scrape preparation.

Basal Cell Carcinoma

Basal cell carcinoma is one of the most common skin tumors, occurring in actinically damaged skin. A definitive diagnosis cannot always be achieved by clinical examination; hence, surgical excision has been used for diagnosis. Cytologic diagnosis is easy and less expensive. The criteria include the presence of the following: (1) tissue fragments with good intercellular cohesion, some with distinct sharp borders; (2) palisading of peripheral cell layer; (3) high nuclear/cytoplasmic ratio in morphologically uniform tumor cells with a thin rim of basophilic cytoplasm; and (4) oval or round nuclei with evenly distributed chromatin and occasional round nucleoli (Fig. 7-27).[42–44]

Squamous Cell Carcinomas

Squamous cell tumors also occur in actinically damaged skin and at mucocutaneous junctions and are cytologically similar to squamous cell carcinomas from other locations.

Malignant Melanomas

Melanomas are divided into four main types, with the superficial spreading and nodular varieties accounting for 70% and 15%, respectively. A small superficial melanoma is an absolute contraindication to FNA and should be diagnosed by excisional biopsy. Large nodular melanomas and recurrent tumors can, however, be diagnosed by FNA. The cytologic features are similar to melanomas in other parts and have been previously described.

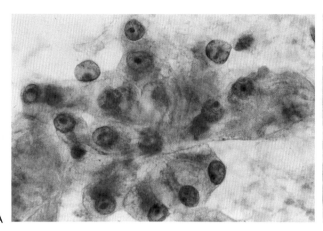 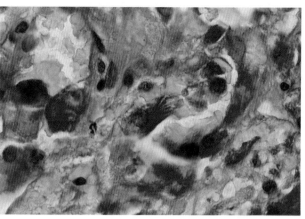

A   B

FIG. 7-26. Alveolar soft part sarcoma. **(A)** Tumor in the soft tissues of the deltoid region demonstrating cells with fragile cytoplasm, round nuclei with prominent nucleoli. (Papanicolaou stain, ×900) **(B)** Periodic acid–Schiff (PAS) stain with diastase digestion demonstrating PAS-positive diastase-resistant crystalloids corresponding to the dark and light filaments seen on electron microscopy. (PAS stain with diastase digestion, ×900)

Melanin pigment can be demonstrated by the Fontana stain. Immunocytochemistry shows S-100 and HMB-45 positivity.

Pilomatrixoma

A pilomatrixoma is a benign adnexal tumor with hair matrix differentiation that usually presents in the first two decades as a dermal or subcutaneous nodule in the head, neck, or upper extremity. Cytologic smears show two types of cells, basophilic and shadow. The basaloid cells are arranged in tight clusters or sheets with poorly defined cell borders, scant cyanophilic cytoplasm, and a high nuclear/cytoplasmic ratio. The nuclei are hyperchromatic and oval to triangular with occasional nuclear molding. Mitotic figures are rare. The shadow cells may be poorly visualized due to the lack of nuclei and slight affinity of the cytoplasm for staining. Well-stained cells possess distinct cell borders, and the keratinized cytoplasm stains brown or yellow on the Papanicolaou stain. A nuclear shadow or clear space is seen in the center of the cell (Fig. 7-28). Nucleated squamous cells, inflammatory cells, calcific deposits, and foreign-body giant cells may be occasionally seen.[45]

Lymphomas

Skin and subcutaneous tissue lymphomas may be primary or a part of disseminated disease. The diagnosis can

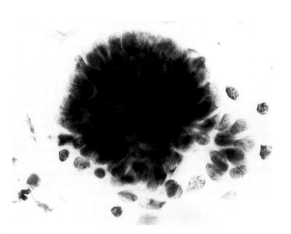

FIG. 7-27. Basal cell carcinoma. Nest of cells with small oval nuclei showing peripheral palisading. (Papanicolaou stain, ×360)

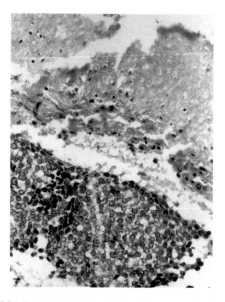

FIG. 7-28. Pilomatrixoma. Small, blue, basaloid cells are seen (*bottom*) adjacent to an epithelial sheet, which consists of "ghosts" of squamous cells, most of which have lost their nuclei (*top*). (Papanicolaou stain, ×360)

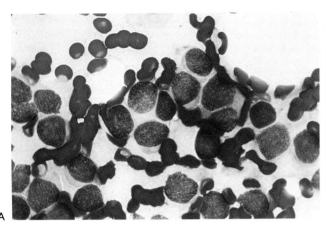
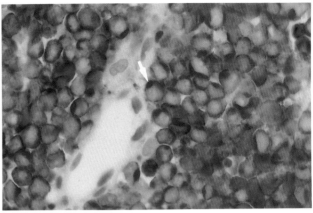

FIG. 7-29. Merkel cell carcinoma. **(A)** Population of small blue cells, with high nuclear/cytoplasmic ratios, obtained from a skin and subcutaneous nodule of the leg in a 90-year-old woman. (Diff-Quik stain, ×900) **(B)** Immunocytochemical stain revealing characteristic keratin positivity. (Keratin, ×360)

be suggested cytologically if a monotonous population of immature lymphoid cells is present. However, histologic confirmation with appropriate marker studies must be performed for a definitive diagnosis.

Merkel Cell Carcinoma

Merkel cell carcinoma usually presents as solitary nodules in the skin of the head and neck. Cytologically, the differential diagnosis is that of a small blue cell tumor, and the diagnosis is made immunocytochemically by the demonstration of the characteristic block pattern of staining with keratin and neuron specific enolase. Electron microscopy demonstrates "dense core" granules (Fig. 7-29).[46-48]

Metastatic Tumors

The most common tumors to metastasize to subcutaneous tissues originate from breast, lung, large intestine, ovaries, stomach, and kidney malignancies. The cytologic features are similar to those of the primary tumor. An example of a metastatic neuroendocrine carcinoma is illustrated in Figure 7-30 and metastatic malignant mixed müllerian tumor in Figure 7-31.

CONCLUSIONS

Although FNA can be helpful to the clinician who is trying to clarify the nature of a soft tissue mass, false results, particularly false-positives, may have serious

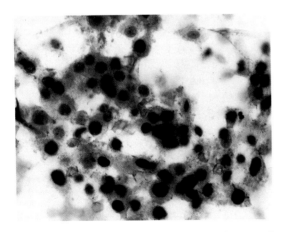

FIG. 7-30. Metastatic neuroendocrine carcinoma. Small, round, blue neoplastic cells with plasmacytoid features and granular cytoplasm. The patient had a history of an islet cell carcinoma that was previously resected. (Papanicolaou stain, ×900)

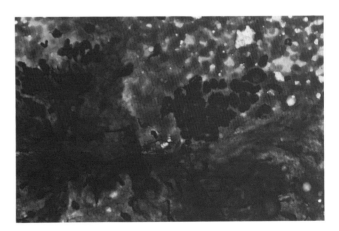

FIG. 7-31. Metastatic malignant mixed müllerian tumor in soft tissues. Aspirate from a periumbilical nodule showing a biphasic pattern consisting of epithelial and stromal elements. The patient had a history of a uterine primary. (Diff-Quik stain, ×900)

effects on management. The reliability of the technique depends on one's ability to interpret the cytomorphologic features of an adequate sample. The cytopathologist should accept some limitations of the technique if adequate sampling is not assured, or the morphology is not well defined because of overlap between some lesions. In such cases, an open biopsy should be recommended.

REFERENCES

1. Wilson RA, Gartner WS. Teflon granuloma mimicking a thyroid tumor. Diagn Cytopathol 1987;3:156.
2. Cavett JR III, McAfee R, Ramzy I. Hansen's disease (leprosy): diagnosis by aspiration biopsy of lymph nodes. Acta Cytol 1986;30:189.
3. Perez-Guillermo M, Hernandez-Gil A, Bonmati C. Diagnosis of cutaneous leishmaniasis by fine needle aspiration cytology. Acta Cytol 1988;32:485.
4. de Boer AL, de Boer F, Van der Merwe JV. Cytologic identification of donovan bodies in granuloma inguinale. Acta Cytol 1984;28:126.
5. Rajwanshi A, Bhambhani S, Das DK. Fine-needle aspiration cytology diagnosis of tuberculosis. Diagn Cytopathol 1987;3:13.
6. Mair S, Leiman G, Levinsohn D. Fine needle aspiration cytology of parotid sarcoidosis. Acta Cytol 1989;33:169.
7. Ramzy I, Rone R, Schantz HD. Squamous cells in needle aspirates of subcutaneous lesions: a diagnostic problem. Am J Clin Pathol 1986;85:319.
8. Oertel YC, Beckner ME, Engler WF. Cytologic diagnosis and ultrastructure of fine-needle aspirates of ganglion cysts. Arch Pathol Lab Med 1986;110:938.
9. Esteban JM, Oertel YC, Mendoza M, et al. Fine needle aspiration in the treatment of ganglion cysts. South Med J 1986;79:691.
10. Peters JL, Thunnissen FBJM, van Heerde P. Fine needle aspiration cytology of radiation-induced changes in nonneoplastic breast lesions. Acta Cytol 1989;33:176.
11. Layfield LJ, Anders KH, Glasgrow BJ, et al. Fine-needle aspiration of primary soft-tissue lesions. Arch Pathol Lab Med 1986;110:420.
12. Wakely PE, Price WG, Frable WJ. Sternomastoid tumor of infancy (fibromatosis colli): diagnosis by aspiration cytology. Mod Pathol 1989;2:37.
13. Griffin JB, Betsill WL. Subcutaneous endometriosis diagnosed by fine needle aspiration cytology. Acta Cytol 1985;29:584.
14. Leiman G, Naylor G. Mucinous metaplasia in scar endometriosis. Diagn Cytopathol 1985;1:153.
15. Bhambhani S, Rajwanski A, Pant L, et al. Fine needle aspiration cytology of supernumerary breast. Acta Cytol 1987;31:311.
16. Orfila C, Giraud P, Modesto A, et al. Abdominal fat tissue aspirate in human amyloidosis. Hum Pathol 1986;17:366.
17. Kanter MH, Duane GB. Angiomatoid malignant fibrous histiocytoma. Arch Pathol Lab Med 1985;109:564.
18. Åkerman M, Rydholm A. Aspiration cytology of intramuscular myxoma. Acta Cytol 1983;27:505.
19. Walaas L, Kindblom LG. Lipomatous tumors: a correlative cytologic and histologic study of 27 tumors examined by fine needle aspiration cytology. Hum Pathol 1985;16:6.
20. Akerman M, Rydholm A. Aspiration cytology of lipomatous tumors: a 10 year experience at an orthopedic oncology center. Diagn Cytopathol 1987;3:295.
21. Abele J, Miller T: Cytology of well-differentiated and poorly differentiated hemangiosarcoma in fine needle aspirates. Acta Cytol 1982;26:341.
22. Gupta RK, Naran S, Dowle C. Needle aspiration cytology and immunocytochemical study in a case of angiosarcoma of the breast. Diagn Cytopathol 1991;7:363.
23. Nguyen GK, McHattie JD, Jeannot A. Cytomorphologic aspects of hepatic angiosarcoma. Acta Cytol 1982;26:527.
24. Perez-Guillermo M, Sola PJ, Garcia RB, et al. FNA cytology of cutaneous vascular tumors. Cytopathology 1992;3:231.
25. Khiyami A, Green L, Georkey F, et al. Primary angiosarcoma of the cuboidal bone: a case report. Diagn Cytopathol 1991;7:520.
26. Young B, Wick M, Fitzgibbon J, et al. CD31 an immunospecific marker for endothelial differentiation in human neoplasms. Appl Immunohistochem 1993;1:97.
27. Sherman M, Joseph D, Gangi M, et al. Immunostaining of small cytologic specimens. Acta Cytol 1994;38:18.
28. Hajdu SI, Hajdu EO. Cytopathology of soft tissue and bone tumors. Basel, Karger, 1989;140.
29. Ramzy I. Benign schwannoma: demonstration of Verocay bodies using fine needle aspiration. Acta Cytol 1977;21:316.
30. Hood IC, Qizilbash AH, Young JEM, et al. Needle aspiration cytology of a benign and a malignant schwannoma. Acta Cytol 1984;28:157.
31. Schwartz JG, Dowd DC. Fine needle aspiration cytology of metastatic malignant schwannoma. Acta Cytol 1988;33:377.
32. Matsuda M, Sone H, Ishiguro S, et al. Fine needle aspiration cytology of malignant schwannoma metastatic to the breast. Acta Cytol 1989;33:372.
33. Fuzes L, Hoer PW, Schmidt W. Exfoliative cytology of multiple endobronchial granular cell tumor. Acta Cytol 1989;33:516.
34. Ogawa K, Nakashima Y, Yamabe H, et al. Alveolar soft part sarcoma, granular cell tumor and paraganglioma. Acta Pathol Jpn 1986;36(Suppl 6):895.
35. Thomas L, Risbud M, Gabriel JB, et al. Cytomorphology of granular-cell tumor of the bronchus. Acta Cytol 1984;28:129.
36. Ordonez NG, Hickey RC, Brooks TE. Alveolar soft part sarcoma. Cancer 1988;61:525.
37. Lieberman PH, Brennan MF, Kimmel M, et al. Alveolar soft-part sarcoma. Cancer 1989;63:1.
38. Mukai M, Torikata C, Iri H, et al. Histogenesis of alveolar soft part sarcoma. Am J Surg Pathol 1986;10:212.
39. Kapila K, Chopra P, Verma K. Fine needle aspiration cytology of alveolar soft-part sarcoma. Acta Cytol 1985;29:559.
40. Brown CL, Klaber MR, Robertson MG. Rapid cytological diagnosis of basal cell carcinoma of the skin. J Clin Pathol 1979;32:361.
41. Slater DN, Reilly G. Fine needle aspiration cytology in dermatology: a clinicopathological appraisal. Br J Dermatol 1986;115:317.
42. Malberger E, Tillinger R, Lichtig C. Diagnosis of basal-cell carcinoma with aspiration cytology. Acta Cytol 1984;28:301.
43. Youngberg GA, Laucirica R, Leicht SS. Frequency of occurrence of diagnostic cytologic parameters in basal cell carcinoma. Am J Clin Pathol 1989;91:24.
44. Bocking A, Schunck K, Auffermann W. Exfoliative-cytologic diagnosis of basal-cell carcinoma, with the use of DNA image cytometry as a diagnostic aid. Acta Cytol 1987;31:143.
45. Solanki P, Ramzy I, Durr N, et al. Pilomatrixoma. Arch Pathol Lab Med 1987;111:294.
46. Mellbolm L, Akerman M, Carlén B. Aspiration cytology of neuroendocrine carcinoma of the skin. Acta Cytol 1984;28:297.
47. Pettinato G, Dechiara A, Insabato L, et al. Neuroendocrine carcinoma of the skin. Acta Cytol 1984;28:283.
48. Spzak C, Bossen E, Linder J, et al. Cytomorphology of primary small cell carcinoma of the skin in fine needle aspirates. Acta Cytol 1984;28:290.
49. Weidner N, Tjoe J. Immunohistochemical profile of monoclonal antibody O13. Am J Surg Pathol 1994;18:486.

Subject Index

ERIALS MUST BE RETURNED
BAR